The Gunn Approach to the
TREATMENT OF CHRONIC PAIN

For Churchill Livingstone

Commissioning Editor: Inta Ozols
Project Manager: Valerie Burgess
Project Editor: Dinah Thom
Design Direction: Judith Wright
Copy Editor: Ruth Swann
Project Controller: Derek Robertson/Pat Miller
Sales Promotion Executive: Maria O'Connor

The Gunn Approach to the
TREATMENT OF CHRONIC PAIN

Intramuscular Stimulation for Myofascial Pain of Radiculopathic Origin

CHURCHILL LIVINGSTONE
An imprint of Elsevier Limited

First Edition 1989
Japanese Edition 1995
Second Edition 1996
    Reprinted 1997, 1999, 2002 (twice), 2003, 2004, 2005, 2007

ISBN 978 0 443 05422 8

British Library Cataloguing in Publication Data
A catalogue record for this book is available from the British Library

Library of Congress Cataloguing in Publication Data
A catalogue record for this book is available from the Library of Congress

your source for books,
journals and multimedia
in the health sciences
www.elsevierhealth.com

Working together to grow
libraries in developing countries

www.elsevier.com | www.bookaid.org | www.sabre.org

ELSEVIER   BOOK AID International   Sabre Foundation

The publisher's policy is to use paper manufactured from sustainable forests

Printed in the United States of America

Transferred to Digital Printing, 2011

Contents

Foreword   ix
Preface to Second Edition   xi
Acknowledgements   xiii
Introduction   xv

PART 1

An overview   1

An introduction to radiculopathic
   pain   3
IMS—the technique   11
Treating chronic pain   17
References for Part 1   18

PART 2

Intramuscular stimulation in
   practice   21

Summary   23
Guidelines for diagnosis   25
Treatment and needle technique   31
General examination   39
Regional examination and specific
   treatment   47
   Cervical spine   51
   Upper limb   61
      Shoulder   61
      Elbow and forearm   66
      Wrist and hand   71
   Back   75
      Dorsal back   75
      Lumbar back   78

Lower limb   87
   Buttock   87
   Posterior thigh   90
   Anterior thigh and knee   91
   Leg and dorsum of foot   96
   Calf   99
   Foot   101

PART 3

Supplementary information   105

Musculoskeletal pain of spondylotic
   origin   107
Table I. Shortened muscles in
   common syndromes   115
Table II. Segmental innervation of
   muscles   117
Sources of supplies   121
Suggested reading   123
Abbreviations for commonly treated
   muscles   125

PART 4

Appendices   127

List of appendices   129

Index   161

UNIVERSITY OF WASHINGTON SCHOOL OF MEDICINE
Seattle, Washington 98105-6920

Dr. Chan Gunn has been a clinical member of the University of Washington Multidisciplinary Pain Center and a consultant at the Center's Pain Clinic since 1983. During this time we have come to value his expertise in diagnosis and treatment of many difficult chronic pain patients. His stimulating and informative teaching sessions have been enjoyed by trainees, staff and visiting physicians on a regular basis adding to the quality of our instruction and patient care. This manual is a thorough and concise guide to diagnosis and therapy as taught by Dr. Gunn.

Dr. Gunn has made significant contributions to the understanding of chronic pain by introducing a theoretical basis which explains many of the enigmatic problems seen in chronic pain clinics. His work has emerged as the end product of his extensive experience with injured workmen. His methods, which can be used in everyday medical practice, are an innovative neurologic approach that yields effective, safe and inexpensive treatment for the many patients who might otherwise remain without pain relief. The importance of his approach can be appreciated if one understands the magnitude of the chronic pain problem and the failures of conventional medicine.

Dr. Gunn considers persisting pain to be the result of subtle dysfunction in the nervous system that often goes unrecognized. His theory is validated by parallel findings and demonstrations by regional anesthesiologic procedures. However, anesthesiologists have limited their work to extreme, and therefore, more dramatic cases and have not applied the same principles to more ordinary, trauma-related injuries. Moreover, their treatments can only be delivered by highly trained regional nerve block specialists, and such treatments carry some risk. Dr. Gunn's independently derived, practical approach can be of great value to a large number of patients with minimal dependence on expensive technology and highly trained specialists.

Like acupuncturists, Dr. Gunn employs needle stimulation without drugs, but his methods are grounded in a solid, physiological conceptual scheme. His theory accounts for the persisting pain and fatigue seen in many patients who suffer for years following a traumatic injury or accident. By using energy (electrical energy, mechanical force, current of needle-induced injury), the therapist using his methods can elicit spinal reflexes and central nervous system responses that promote healing, and more important, rehabilitation. His procedures are a viable alternative to the prescription of drugs, which foster toxicity, and to surgery which all too often causes more harm than benefit.

We enthusiastically recommend this manual to all practitioners dealing with chronic pain, to aid in diagnosis and therapy of complex pain problems.

John D. Loeser MD
Professor, Neurological Surgery & Anesthesiology
Director, Multidisciplinary Pain Center

C. Richard Chapman PhD
Professor Anesthesiology,
Psychiatry and Behavioral Sciences
and Psychology

Stephen Butler MD
Associate Professor
Anesthesiology

Anders E. Sola MD
Clinical Assistant Professor
Anesthesiology

Myofascial pain syndromes plague both patients and those who try to provide relief. Criteria for diagnosis and treatment have not been widely accepted; outcome studies are few. Most of our successes have come from the dedicated efforts of a small number of physicians who have made myofascial pains the subjects of their lives' work. My friend and colleague, Chan Gunn, has been one of the most creative and successful practitioners in this vexatious field. He has not only developed a useful conceptual framework that explains the physical findings but also has perfected a simple and effective treatment technique. Although this book summarizes his thoughts and treatment techniques, it cannot begin to be as useful as a learning tool as observing Chan Gunn examine and treat a patient. I am delighted that the First Edition of his text has now been translated into Japanese so our colleagues in that country can learn of his methods. Dr. Gunn has greatly enriched the treatment of patients at the University of Washington Multidisciplinary Pain Center; those who read and master this book will be able to bring effective pain relief to their patients.

John D. Loeser MD
Director, Multidisciplinary Pain Center
Professor, Neurological Surgery and Anesthesiology

Foreword

I consider this book to be in the best of the traditions of classical medicine. Its start point is a profound understanding of the anatomy and physiology of movement and of inability to move. The author describes this in the terms which have been used by clinicians throughout this century and proceeds to describe methods of diagnostic examination with the intention of giving a precise location to the centre of the disorder. For this he uses the most sensitive of tools, the eyes and hands of an intelligent trained observer. Finally, in the third stage he disturbs the environment of the disordered site in an empirical and exactly described manner. He observes that this intrusion into a defined area in a defined manner is followed by an alleviation of signs and symptoms.

I would strongly object if anyone labelled this procedure as being complementary or alternative to traditional medicine. There are three reasons to recognise its traditional nature. His method of diagnosis and description of the disorder is based entirely on generally accepted factors in anatomy, physiology and pathology, without any introduction of mystical forces or energies which characterise so much of what is called alternative medicine. It is true that he characterises the precise nature of the disorders in terms of neuropathies and compressions, but these are hypotheses which are permissible because they are testable by accepted methods of investigation. Almost all traditional medical and surgical diagnoses and therapies are based on hypotheses which have not yet been fully tested and proven. Secondly, the fact that he uses needles does not mean that he does so for the mystical unproven reasons on which Chinese acupuncture is based. After all, it was Helen Travell MD who introduced the phrase he uses, "dry needling", when she discovered in the course of injecting local anaesthetic into tender points that it was not necessary to inject the local anaesthetic, since it was the insertion of the needle which produced the effect. Lastly, the therapeutic effect is open for exact scientific observation, analysis and test. It is in order to encourage this last fraction that this book is written. Gunn attempts here to define in a teachable manner the diagnosis and the therapy. Elsewhere he is setting up an institute for training and for investigation.

I also think it would be unwise to pick out one aspect from the broad background of Dr. Gunn to highlight the importance of this book. It is true that he is of Chinese-Malaysian origin and is therefore familiar with the great tradition of Chinese medicine. However, his own educational background could not be more Western and traditional with his medical degree from Cambridge, his residency training in medicine and surgery, and his extensive clinical experience in family medicine and in industrial medicine. This is a highly intelligent observant man who is surely affected by many factors simultaneously.

Finally, I hope that the reader will take this book as a very serious challenge and not a simple easy recipe. First, it requires a meticulous hands-on clinical examination of the individual patient. This itself is becoming a lost art in favour of supposedly effective high-tech methods. Secondly, it requires subtle sensitive empirical treatment of the individual patient. Third, it requires analysis and recording of the patient's reaction. This book is not an authoritative patriarchal set of orders. It encourages the reader to take the experience of one apparently effective therapist and to explore from that start point.

P.D.W.

Preface to Second Edition

Chronic myofascial pain—or pain that occurs in the musculoskeletal system without any obvious cause—often defies treatment. Medications and commonly available physical therapies usually give only temporary relief. Many patients, therefore, wander from therapist to therapist in a vain quest for relief.

This practical manual explains Intramuscular Stimulation (IMS), a comprehensive, alternative system of diagnosis and treatment which was first developed and proven at the Workers' Compensation Board of British Columbia. IMS is now taught and employed at the University of Washington's Multidisciplinary Pain Center at Seattle, Washington. From Seattle, trained pain Fellows have taken IMS back to their home countries all over the world. A Japanese edition was published in June 1995. The success of this technique has led to a new model for chronic pain which was presented to the Royal College of Physicians and Surgeons of Canada in 1985 (Appendix 1).

The manual is directed at general practitioners, orthopedic and sports medicine physicians, anesthesiologists and rheumatologists and others who seek a more effective physical modality for the management of chronic myofascial pain.

Myofascial pain is typically accompanied by sensory, motor and autonomic manifestations that indicate some functional disturbances and/or pathological changes in the peripheral nervous system—that is, neuropathy. A large number of chronic pain syndromes belong to this category of pain; this is sometimes called neuropathic pain, but because, in our experience, neuropathy occurs almost always at the nerve root, "radiculopathic pain" is a more accurate term.

Myofascial pain syndromes can occur in any part of the body and are customarily considered as distinct and unrelated local conditions (e.g. "lateral epicondylitis", "bicipital tendonitis", and so on). But since pain and neuropathic manifestations in all of these conditions respond to the same type of treatment regardless of the location of the pain, the underlying mechanism is the same, wherever the syndrome may present. Thus, there may be hundreds of "conditions", but only one cause—radiculopathy. In radiculopathy, signs are found in the distribution of both primary rami of the segmental nerve. Frequently, pain persists unless muscles belonging to both rami—especially paraspinal muscles—are treated.

The causes of neuropathy are numerous, but clinical findings, as described in this manual, indicate that spondylosis (the structural disintegration and morphologic alterations that occur in the intervertebral disc with pathoanatomic changes in surrounding structures), which is near-universal, is the most common cause (Appendix 2).

A crucial ingredient of myofascial

pain is muscle shortening from contractures. In fact, myofascial pain does not exist without shortening. Prolonged muscle shortening can not only cause pain in muscle, it also mechanically pulls on tendons, thereby straining them and distressing the joints they act on. The increased wear and tear in joints eventually leads to degenerative changes (e.g. "osteoarthritis").

The goal of treatment is to release muscle shortening. Unfortunately, commonly used physical therapies are often ineffective in chronic conditions: a needle technique is then necessary. Medications may be injected, but the use of a needle without injected substances, or "dry needling", is just as effective. Intramuscular stimulation is a special application of dry needling.

Our system of IMS is based on neurophysiologic concepts, but the technique and implements for needling are borrowed from traditional acupuncture. Unlike acupuncture, however, IMS requires a medical examination and diagnosis and treats points that are specific anatomic entities selected according to physical signs.

In recent years, the injection of "trigger points" has become widely used. Our system has features in common with the trigger point approach but differs in concept and objectives. The trigger point approach regards painful points primarily as localized phenomena—foci of hyperirritable tissue (myofascial, cutaneous, fascial, ligamentous, and periosteal) occurring as the result of compensatory overload, shortened range, or response to activity in other trigger points. Instead, we view pain as only one of several possible manifestations or epiphenomena of radiculopathy. (Dysfunction occurs also in the other components of the segmental nerve—motor, sensory, and autonomic.) In trigger point therapy, focal sources of noxious input are eliminated by therapy directed primarily to the affected muscles. In our concept, needling not only produces local inflammation which is the necessary prelude to healing, but also influences distant components of the segmental nerve by reflex stimulation. For example, it can relax shortening in smooth muscles (in blood vessels and viscera). Furthermore, because neural dysfunction occurs as the result of radiculopathy, a prime purpose of IMS treatment is to relieve shortening in paraspinal muscles that entraps the nerve root and perpetuates pain.

Our needle technique is safe **in qualified hands,** and has few iatrogenic side-effects. It is effective in chronic musculoskeletal pain when muscle shortening resists conventional physical therapies. The technique is also unequaled for finding muscle shortening in deep muscles that are normally inaccessible to the palpating finger.

Those interested in using IMS may acquire basic needling techniques by joining their local medical acupuncture society. For a practical demonstration of IMS, contact the University of Washington's Multidisciplinary Pain Center, Seattle, or the author at Gunn Pain Clinic, 828 West Broadway, Vancouver, British Columbia, Canada V5Z 1J8; telephone 1 (604) 873-4866. An introductory video-recording of the technique is also available.

Seattle 1996   C.C.G.

Acknowledgements

John D. Loeser MD
President, International Association for the
Study of Pain
Director, Multidisciplinary Pain Center
Professor, Neurological Surgery and
Anesthesiology University of Washington

Thomas F. Hornbein MD
Professor and Former Chairman,
Anesthesiology; Professor,
Physiology and Biophysics, University of
Washington

C. Richard Chapman PhD
Professor, Anesthesiology, Psychiatry &
Behavioral Sciences, and Psychology,
University of Washington
Director, Pain and Toxicity Research Program,
Fred Hutchinson Cancer Research Center,
Seattle

Stephen H. Butler MD
Associate Professor, Anesthesiology, University
of Washington

F. Peter Buckley MB BS FFARCS
Associate Professor, Anesthesiology, University
of Washington

Anders E. Sola MD
Clinical Assistant Professor, Anesthesiology,
University of Washington

Mathew Lee MD
American College of Acupuncture

Bengt Johansson MD
Chairman, Swedish Association of Orthopedic
Medicine

Acupuncture Foundation of Canada

American Academy of Acupuncture

**British Medical Acupuncture
Society**

**Physical Medicine Research
Foundation**

**Health Science Center for
Educational Resources**
John R. Bolles, Assistant Director
Auriel Clare, Editor
Kate Sweeney, Medical Illustrator

M. Kitihara MD, Editor of the Japanese
Edition

Introduction

WHAT IS INTRAMUSCULAR STIMULATION (IMS)?

- Intramuscular stimulation, or IMS, is a total system for the diagnosis and treatment of myofascial pain syndromes (chronic pain conditions that occur in the musculoskeletal system when there is no obvious injury or inflammation).
- IMS explains this large category of pain in a new way. Instead of presuming pain to be signals of tissue injury, IMS blames pain on unwell nerves (when there is disturbed function and supersensitivity in the peripheral nervous system—"neuropathic pain").
- IMS applies Cannon and Rosenblueth's law of denervation to explain the supersensitivity that occurs with peripheral neuropathy. This physiologic law is fundamental but little known.
- IMS has introduced an examination technique that shows neuropathy to occur, almost invariably, at the nerve root—causing "radiculopathic pain". Because there is no satisfactory laboratory or imaging test for neuropathy, IMS's clinical examination is indispensable for diagnosis.
- IMS's radiculopathy model explains many apparently different and unrelated pain syndromes—from headache to low back pain, from tennis elbow to trigeminal neuralgia—and places them all into one classification.
- IMS borrows its needle technique from traditional Chinese acupuncture, but updates and enhances it with anatomy and neurophysiology. IMS is simple to learn for doctors, nurses and therapists who have training in anatomy. Results are predictable and superior to acupuncture because treatment is based on physical signs.
- IMS should be taught in medical schools because it is more effective than any other physical therapy. Knowledge of IMS can provide an excellent bridge between Eastern and Western medicine. Indeed, not only does IMS bridge the gap between them, it transcends the limitations of both.

HOW INTRAMUSCULAR STIMULATION DEVELOPED

IMS and the radiculopathy model was developed from clinical observations and research carried out over a period of more than twenty years—first, at the Workers' Compensation Board of British Columbia and, subsequently, at my pain clinic in Vancouver.

IMS began in 1973. Frustrated by the generally unsatisfactory results obtained when using conventional physical therapies for chronic pain patients, I needed to learn more about chronic pain. I therefore carefully examined 100 patients who had chronic back pain but who did not have obvious signs of injury, and 100 controls who did not have pain. The significant finding was that patients who were disabled for a long period had tenderness in muscles belonging to affected myotomes. *Tender points are therefore sensitive indicators of radicular involvement and differentiate a simple mechanical low back strain (which usually heals quickly) from one with neural involvement which is slow to improve* (Appendix 3).

My next study of 50 patients with "tennis elbow" showed that tender points at the elbow were related to cervical spondylosis and radiculopathy. *Treating the neck, but not the elbow, provided relief* (Appendix 4).

A study of pain in the shoulder similarly implicated radiculopathy in the cervical spine (Appendix 5).

Further careful examination of patients with chronic pain revealed additional signs of radiculopathy. *A pattern began to emerge—patients who have pain, but no obvious signs of injury, generally have subtle but discernible signs of peripheral nerve involvement.* This is an important observation because there is no satisfactory laboratory or imaging test for early neural dysfunction. IMS's method of examination is now recommended as part of the evaluation process in Bonica's textbook *The Management of Pain*.

Medical diagnosis traditionally assumes that pain is a signal of injury or inflammation conveyed to the CNS via healthy nerves. However, our studies have led us to conclude that pain can arise, when there is no injury or inflammation, from radiculopathy that accompanies incipient spondylosis (Appendix 2— this paper was determined as a significant study by the 1979 Volvo Competition Awards Committee). The term "neuropathic pain" has

been given to this category of pain, but because neuropathy is almost invariably at the nerve root, "radiculopathic" pain is a more appropriate name.

I became interested in acupuncture in 1974. An early observation was that most acupuncture points correspond to known neuroanatomic entities, such as muscle motor points or musculotendinous junctions.

Traditional acupuncturists emphasize the importance of producing the subjective sensation of *Teh Ch'i* or *Deqi* when the needle penetrates muscle and is grasped by a contracture. Failure of a needle to produce needle-grasp signifies that the muscle is not shortened and will not respond to needle treatment. Traditional Chinese medicine has long recognised that *this category of chronic pain is never present without associated muscle shortening from contracture.*

We tested dry needling in a randomized clinical trial but, unlike traditional Chinese acupuncture, in our approach (which was the beginning of IMS) patients were needled at muscle motor points. The group that had been treated with needling was found to be significantly better than the control group (Appendix 6). (This clinical trial was also determined as a significant study by the 1979 Volvo Competition Awards Committee.)

A paper proposing that causalgia is a manifestation of denervation supersensitivity was read at the 1979 meeting of the International Association for the Study of Pain (IASP).

An interesting observation in patients with neuropathic pain was the finding of hair loss in affected dermatomes. If treatment is given early and effectively, hair sometimes returns. We wondered whether a deficit of the trophic factor was to blame, and whether there is a similar deficit of the factor in male pattern hair loss (Appendix 7).

IMS differs from traditional acupuncture in that it:

- requires a medical examination using our early signs of radiculopathy
- requires a medical diagnosis that implicates spondylosis
- uses neuroanatomic points that are found in a radicular or segmental pattern, instead of using traditional acupuncture points
- determines the points to be treated; the effects of needling can appear very quickly and progress can be monitored through objective physical signs.

Our conclusion is that muscle shortening, autonomic changes, and sometimes pain, are natural occurrences and epiphenomena of radiculopathy (Appendix 1), and they all occur according to Cannon and Rosenblueth's law of denervation. Our radiculopathy model is able to explain many puzzling chronic pains that are not caused by injury or inflammation, such as low back pain, tennis elbow, whiplash and fibromyalgia (Appendix 8).

COMPARING ACUPUNCTURE TO IMS	
Acupuncture	**IMS**
Medical diagnosis not relevant	Medical diagnosis necessary
Medical examination not applicable	Medical examination imperative
Needle insertions according to Chinese philosophy into non-scientific meridians	Needle insertions as indicated by examination, e.g. muscle motor points
Knowledge of anatomy not applicable	Knowledge of anatomy essential
No immediate objective changes anticipated	Prompt subjective and objective effects often expected

Part I

An overview

An introduction to radiculopathic pain

WHAT IS PAIN?

What is pain? The definition of pain given by the International Association for the Study of Pain is: "an unpleasant sensory and emotional experience associated with actual or potential tissue damage, or described by the patient in terms of such damage".

This definition can be misleading because pain is not just one, but at least three distinct entities—immediate, acute, and chronic.[43] Furthermore, pain, which is the central perception of noxious input, can arise from non-painful signals that are misperceived as painful ones. Pain can even arise when there is no external input—radiculopathic pain is a common example.

THE THREE PHASES OF PAIN. WHICH RESPONDS TO IMS?

Pain is a general reaction pattern of three distinct, sequential, and natural behavioral phases: immediate, acute, and chronic.[43] Immediate pain, or nociception, is the prompt signalling of tissue threat or damage via injury-sensitive A-delta and C fibers, but persistent nociception is not a common cause of chronic pain.[2,47] Inflammation can generate acute pain by producing algogenic substances that activate nociceptors (e.g. histamine, bradykinin, prostaglandins, and others), but inflammation is easily recognized by pain, redness, increased local temperature, and swelling. Furthermore, inflammation is usually self-limiting, unless there is an abnormal immunologic response as in rheumatoid arthritis.[24]

Chronic pain can occur if any of the following are present:
- Ongoing nociception or inflammation.
- Psychologic factors such as a somatization disorder, depression, or operant learning processes.
- Functional and structural alterations within the central or peripheral nervous systems.[2]

The term neuropathic pain has been applied to the last category (Appendix 2).[10] Neuropathic pain often arises and persists indefinitely in the absence of a detectable permanent injury or inflammation. Such pain seems a paradox—a response occurs and is sustained without a discernible stimulus. IMS has unique applicability in musculoskeletal pain syndromes belonging to this category of chronic pain.

CHRONIC MUSCULOSKELETAL PAIN OF NEUROPATHIC ORIGIN: ITS RELATIONSHIP TO RADICULOPATHY

Myofascial pain syndromes are mundane, and can affect joints, muscles, and their connective tissue attachments in all parts of the body. Because their clinical presentations are diverse, they are customarily identified as separate and unrelated conditions, and typically labelled according to the painful part, e.g. "lateral epicondylitis", "Achilles tendonitis", etc. (see Table I).

However, most musculoskeletal pain syndromes are accompanied by sensory, motor and autonomic findings that indicate some functional disturbances and/or pathological changes in the peripheral nerves (i.e. neuropathy). These neuropathic findings generally occur in the distribution of both dorsal and ventral rami of segmental nerves, i.e. radiculopathy. Much less commonly, the distribution is that of a mononeuropathy.

Since pain and other manifestations are, in fact, epiphenomena of radiculopathy, they appear and also resolve in unison following treatment. They have their common origin in some functional dysfunction of the peripheral nervous system and pain may be the result of abnormal nerve connections and/or spurious activity in the pain sensory system.[1,8,10,21,31,32,40,44,45]

CAUSES OF NEUROPATHY: SPONDYLOSIS IS THE MOST COMMON CAUSE

The causes of neuropathy are as numerous as those of nerve damage, and may include neoplasm, toxicity, inflammation, trauma, and vascular, metabolic, infectious, and degenerative changes.[4] The peripheral nervous system is more susceptible to damage than the central nervous system: the spinal root within the spinal canal and intervertebral foramina, and after it emerges, is especially vulnerable.[46] (Even in a peripheral lesion such as carpal tunnel syndrome, there may be an associated entrapment of the nerve root.[42])

Attrition to the nerve root may result from a number of mechanisms, including pressure, stretch, angulation, and friction. Spondylosis (the structural disintegration and morphologic alterations that occur in the intervertebral disc, with pathoanatomic changes in surrounding structures) can precipitate and aggravate these mechanisms. Since spondylosis is near-universal, it is by far the most common cause of radiculopathy. Our clinical findings as described in this manual support this. Other causes of radiculopathy such as arachnoiditis, neuroma, and intraspinal tumors are much less common.[4]

Ordinarily, spondylosis follows a gradual, relapsing, and remitting course that is silent, unless and until symptoms are precipitated by an incident often so minor that it passes unnoticed by the patient. All gradations of spondylosis can exist, but early or incipient spondylotic changes, even when unsuspected, can cause radiculopathy (Appendix 2).

Our emphasis on radiculopathy is not without reason: with an acute injury to a healthy nerve, there is no prolonged discharge of pain signals, whereas the same injury to a neuropathic nerve can cause a sustained discharge. In other words, for pain to become a persistent symptom, the affected fibers must be previously irritated or defective. That is why some people develop severe pain after an apparently minor injury, and why that pain can continue beyond a "reasonable" period.

Spondylosis increases with age, therefore spondylotic pain is more common in middle-aged individuals who have accumulated what Sola has termed an "injury pool"—an accumulation of repeated major and minor injuries to a segment leading to unresolved clinical residuals which may, or may not, produce pain.[35]

CLINICAL FEATURES OF NEUROPATHIC PAIN

Neuropathic pain is distinguished by:
- Pain in the absence of an ongoing tissue-damaging process.
- Delay in onset after precipitating injury.
- Abnormal or unpleasant sensations such as "burning or searing" pain (dysesthesia), or "deep, aching" pain which is more common than dysesthetic pain in musculoskeletal pain syndromes.
- Pain felt in a region of sensory deficit.
- Paroxysmal brief "shooting or stabbing" pain.
- A mild stimulus causing extreme pain (allodynia).
- Pronounced summation and after-reaction with repetitive stimuli.
- Loss of joint range or pain caused by the mechanical effects of muscle shortening.

Any of the above features should raise the suspicion of neuropathic pain.[1,10]

Neuropathy is determined principally by clinical examination as there can be nerve dysfunction without any detectable structural changes. Most clinical neuropathies are of mixed pathology; both axonal degeneration and segmental demyelination can occur in varying degrees.[4]

Routine laboratory and radiological tests are unhelpful,[10] but may be indicated, e.g.: electromyography (EMG) to determine primary disease of muscle; radiology to exclude intraspinal tumors; and laboratory investigations to rule out abnormal immunologic response. EMG, before denervation, may only show increased insertion activity, and nerve conduction velocities can be normal, but F-wave latencies may be prolonged.[4,38] Thermography may reveal altered skin temperature but does not, by itself, indicate pain.[39]

Radiological findings of spinal degenerative changes, commonplace in the middle-aged, should not be dismissed as they can imply some degree of previous nerve damage.

RADICULOPATHIC DYSFUNCTION

Neuropathy is most often at root level (i.e. radiculopathy) when mixed sensory, motor and autonomic disturbances which are epiphenomena of radiculopathy will present in the dermatomal, myotomal, and sclerotomal target structures supplied by the segmental nerve. They are often symmetrical; even when symptoms are unilateral, latent signs may be mirrored contralaterally.[10,14,18]

Dysfunction need not include pain unless nociceptive pathways are involved: some neuropathies are pain-free,[38] such as sudomotor hyper-activity in hyperhidrosis, and muscle weakness in ventral root disease.

If and when pain is present, it is practically always accompanied by:

- muscle shortening in peripheral and paraspinal muscles
- tender and painful focal areas in muscles ("trigger points")[14,15,33,35,36,41]
- autonomic and trophic manifestations of neuropathy.[28,38,41]

CANNON AND ROSENBLUETH'S LAW OF DENERVATION

Normal nerve and muscle depend

upon intact innervation to provide a regulatory or "trophic" effect. Formerly, it was supposed that loss of the trophic factor, through total denervation, led to "denervation supersensitivity". More recently, it has been shown that any measure which blocks the flow of motor impulses and deprives the effector organ of excitatory input for a period of time can cause "disuse supersensitivity" in that organ, as well as in associated spinal reflexes. "Supersensitive" nerves and innervated structures react abnormally to stimuli according to Cannon and Rosenblueth's law of denervation:

When a unit is destroyed, in a series of efferent neurons, an increased irritability to chemical agents develops in the isolated structure or structures, the effect being maximal in the part directly denervated.

In other words, when a nerve is below par and is not functioning properly (neuropathy), it becomes supersensitive and will behave erratically. This principle is fundamental and universal, yet it is not at all well known or credited!

Cannon and Rosenblueth recognized four types of increased sensitivity: the amplitude of response is unchanged but its time-course is prolonged (super-duration of response); the threshold of the stimulating agent is lower than normal (hyperexcitability); lessened stimuli which do not have to exceed a threshold produce responses of normal amplitude (increased susceptibility); and, the capacity of the tissue to respond is augmented (superreactivity).

They also demonstrated that supersensitivity can occur in many structures of the body including skeletal muscle, smooth muscle, spinal neurons, sympathetic ganglia, adrenal glands, sweat glands, and even brain cells. Furthermore, they showed that denervated structures overreact to a wide variety of chemical and physical inputs including stretch and pressure.

THE SHORTENED MUSCLE SYNDROME

Of all the structures that develop supersensitivity, the most common and significant is striated muscle. Apart from pain and tenderness that may occur within muscle (possibly from the compression of supersensitive nociceptors), neuropathy increases muscle tone and causes concurrent muscle shortening. Muscle shortening, in turn, can mechanically cause a large variety of pain syndromes by its relentless pull on various structures.

Muscle shortening is the key to myofascial pain of neuropathic origin. Stated differently, myofascial pain cannot exist in absence of muscle shortening—no shortening, no pain. We therefore sometimes refer to myofascial pain as the "shortened muscle syndrome".

Muscle shortening, "spasm" and contracture

Muscle shortening is a fundamental feature of musculoskeletal pain syndromes.

The term "spasm" is commonly used to describe muscle shortening in myofascial pain syndromes, but shortening is generally caused by classic contracture. Spasm—that is, increased muscle tension with (or without) muscle shortening—comes from non-voluntary motor nerve activity and is seen in electromyography as continuous motor unit activity. Spasm cannot be stopped by voluntary relaxation. However, EMG examination of a shortened muscle rarely reveals any motor unit activity.

Classic *contracture*, on the other hand, is the evoked shortening of a muscle fiber in the absence of action potentials. In denervated, supersensitive skeletal muscle fibers, acetylcholine slowly depolarizes muscle membrane, and thus induces electromechanical coupling with the consequent slow development of tension without action potentials. Since no action potentials are revealed by electromyography, muscle shortening is most likely caused by contracture.

It is therefore best to avoid using the term "spasm" when describing muscle shortening. (It has recently been suggested that there is direct sympathetic innervation to the intrafusal fibers of muscle spindles and sympathetic stimulation can cause muscle tension in curarized animals that is blocked by alpha-adrenergic antagonists.[21])

Muscle shortening can be palpated as ropey bands within muscle. The bands are seldom limited to a few individual muscles, but are present in groups of muscles according to the pattern of the neuropathy. In radiculopathy, bands are also present in paraspinal muscles.

Secondary pain caused by muscle shortening

An important source of pain in musculoskeletal pain syndromes is from muscle shortening that mechanically stresses muscle attachments, causing conditions such as "bicipital tendonitis" or "lateral epicondylitis".

Shortening in muscles acting across a joint increases joint pressure, upsets alignment, and can precipitate pain in the joint, i.e. arthralgia. Increased pressure upon spinal joints can cause the "facet-joint syndrome". Muscle shortening can eventually bring about degenerative changes—osteoarthritis.

Shortened paraspinal muscles perpetuate radiculopathy by compressing the disc

Shortening in paraspinal muscles acting across a disc space compresses the disc and can cause narrowing of the intervertebral foramina, indirectly irritating the nerve root (e.g. through pressure of a bulging disc), or by direct pressure on the root after it emerges.

A self-perpetuating circle can arise: pressure on a nerve root causes neuropathy; neuropathy leads to pain and shortening in target muscles, including paraspinal muscles; shortening in paraspinal muscles further compresses the nerve root. (This self-perpetuating circle is not the repudiated vicious circle of pain, pressure on blood vessels leading to ischaemia and more pain.)

PAIN IN MUSCLES

Muscle bands are usually pain-free, but can become tender and painful, possibly by compressing intramuscular nociceptors or microneuromas (Appendix 3). Focal areas of tenderness and pain are often referred to as "trigger points". When pain is primarily in muscles and is associated with multiple tender trigger points, the condition is referred to as myofascial pain syndrome.[33,34,35,36,41]

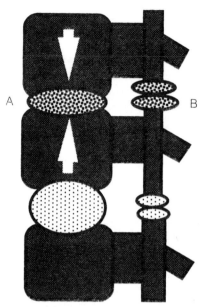

When muscles across a disc shorten, they compress it (A), and at the same time, cause arthralgia in the facet joints (B).

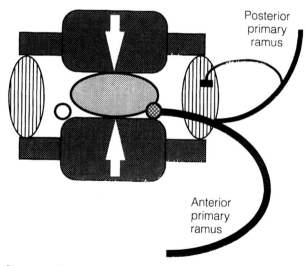

Posterior primary ramus

Anterior primary ramus

Shortened intrinsic back muscles have compressed the disc and impinged on the nerve root. The irritated root further shortens muscles in both rami, thus further irritating the nerve root.

When muscle bands are fibrotic and painful, the condition is sometimes known as "fibrositis", "fibromyalgia", "fibromyositis", or "diffuse myofascial pain syndrome". The etiology of the syndrome is "unknown", but it has many clinical features of the radiculopathic group: pain and stiffness of long duration (> 3 months) increased by physical or mental stress (the role of anxiety and emotional stress in causing muscle spasm and pain is well known); multiple tender points; nerve compression and disc degeneration; soft tissue swelling; joint pain; and neuropathy.[29] (See below.)

AUTONOMIC MANIFESTATIONS OF NEUROPATHY

Autonomic changes are:

- vasomotor
- sudomotor
- pilomotor.

Vasoconstriction generally differentiates neuropathic pain from inflammatory pain; with neuropathic pain, affected parts are perceptibly colder, and retained catabolites from ischemia may exacerbate the pain.[5] There may be increased sudomotor activity, and the pilomotor reflex is often hyperactive and visible in affected dermatomes ("goose-bumps").[15,32]

There can be interaction between pain and autonomic phenomena. A stimulus such as chilling, which excites the pilomotor response, can precipitate pain; vice versa, pressure upon a tender motor point can provoke the pilomotor and sudomotor reflexes.

Increased tone in lymphatic vessel smooth muscle, and increased permeability in blood vessels[37] can

SURFACE EMG AND MYOFASCIAL PAIN

Mark D. Gilbert MD and Heather Tick MD

Surface EMG can measure gross muscle fiber power and demonstrate fatigue and asymmetrical recruitment in myofascial pain syndromes. The typical myofascial pain patient presents sEMG evidence of one or more inhibited muscles. We have witnessed direct evidence of muscle amplitude improvement immediately after IMS needling. The figure shows asymmetry in the scalene muscles and demonstrates change in the EMG signal when a needle is inserted into the right scalene muscle (see arrow). Note the sudden rise in amplitude. The patient noted a significant increase in neck range of motion after this procedure.

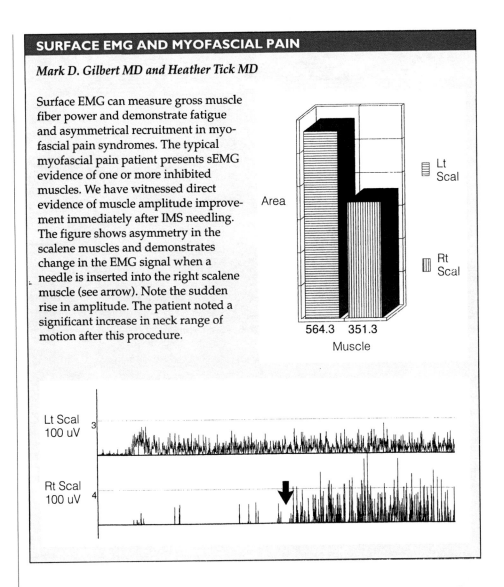

lead to local subcutaneous tissue edema ("neurogenic" edema or "trophedema") (see p. 26). This can be confirmed by the peau d'orange effect (orange peel skin) or by the "Matchstick" test: trophedema is non-pitting to digital pressure, but when a blunt instrument such as the end of a matchstick is used, the indentation produced is clear-cut and persists for minutes.[15] This simple test for neuropathy is more sensitive than electromyography. Trophic changes such as dermatomal hair loss may also accompany neuropathy.

COLLAGEN DEGRADATION

Neuropathy and denervation affect the quality of collagen in soft and skeletal tissues. This is an important factor in chronic pain and degenerative conditions because replacement collagen has fewer cross-links and is markedly weaker than normal

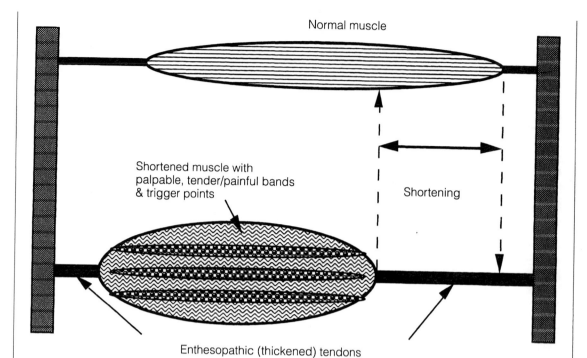

Normal muscle

Shortened muscle with palpable, tender/painful bands & trigger points

Shortening

Enthesopathic (thickened) tendons

mature collagen.[26] Any form of stress —whether emotional or physical, whether extrinsic or intrinsic— causes muscle shortening. The increased mechanical tension that muscle shortening generates hastens wear and tear because it pulls on degraded collagen that provides the strength of ligaments, tendons, cartilage, and bone. Neuropathy expedites degeneration in weight-bearing and activity-stressed parts of the body, causing "spondylosis", "discogenic disease", and "osteo-arthritis" among others. Such conditions are currently regarded as primary diseases, but they are secondary to a radiculopathic process. Radiculopathic pain conditions must therefore be treated with some urgency.

IMS—the technique

Neuropathic pain affects all target structures innervated by the nerve, including joints, muscles, and their connective tissue attachments. While pain may present primarily in a muscle (e.g. shortening in the tibialis anterior muscle causing "shin splints"), or in a tendon (e.g. shortening of the biceps brachii muscle straining its tendon and producing "bicipital tendonitis"), or in a joint (e.g. shortening of the quadriceps femoris muscles giving rise to knee joint pain), all target structures are affected to varying degrees, and the common perpetrator of pain in all these structures is muscle shortening.

We have found that muscle shortening can be released when painful trigger points in the muscle are desensitized. Invariably, when muscle shortening is relieved, pain, whether in muscle, tendon, or joint, is alleviated.

The most effective way to desensitize painful points is to use an intramuscular technique. Injections of local anesthetic, with or without steroids, or saline, may be used; however, injections of medication, especially steroids, can cause side-effects such as infection, impaired healing, weakened tissue elements, local atrophy of fatty tissue and "dimpling" of skin, skin pigmentation, inflammation due to crystal deposits, suppression of the hypothalamic-pituitary axis, localized bleeding, accidental pneumothorax, and joint destruction by avascular necrosis that sometimes imitates a Charcot joint. By contrast, IMS dry needling, which is more effective, has few iatrogenic side-effects (minor localized bleeding and accidental pneumothorax).[27] We prefer IMS dry needling for all of these reasons and others as described below.

NEEDLE TECHNIQUE

The technique of inserting a needle is simple, but good results require a correct diagnosis, a knowledge of muscle anatomy, and practice, especially to accurately reach deep muscle points. We use a fine solid needle (30 gauge or less), usually 1 or 2 inches long, in a plunger-type needle holder. The plunger allows the length of the needle to be varied according to the thickness of the muscle treated. The pointed tip of the solid needle is less traumatic than the beveled, cutting edge of a hollow needle; its flexible and springy quality, unlike that of a rigid hollow needle, transmits the nature and consistency of tissues penetrated. When it enters normal muscle, the needle meets with little resistance;

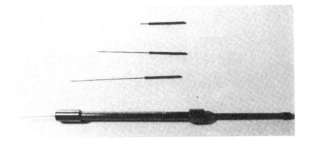

when it pierces a spasm, there is firm resistance, and the needle is "grasped" by the spasm; when it encounters fibrotic tissue, there is grating resistance (like cutting through a pear), and sometimes, when fibrosis is extensive, considerable effort with repeated "pecking" is required. The fine solid needle therefore allows multiple, closely-spaced penetrations to be made without excessive tissue damage, and its whippy nature relays useful feedback information.

Penetration of a shortened muscle can occasionally actuate muscle to fasciculation; this is usually accompanied by near-instantaneous muscle relaxation. Any spasm not thus released invariably grasps the needle, and this can be clearly perceived as the spasm resists the needle's withdrawal.[17] Leaving the grasped needle in situ for a further period (10–20 minutes), generally leads to the needle's release and to pain relief. *Failure to induce needle-grasp signifies that muscle shortening is not the cause of pain and that the condition would probably not respond to this type of treatment.* Penetration into almost any part of the muscle can lead to relaxation, but the most rewarding sites are at tender and painful points in muscle bands. These points (which often correspond to traditional acupuncture points[19,30]) are generally situated beneath muscle motor points, and at musculo-tendinous junctions.

THE "TEH CH'I" PHENOMENON OR "DEQI"

Subjectively, penetrating into a normal muscle is nearly painless, but when a contracture is encountered the patient experiences a peculiar, cramp-like sensation as the needle is grasped. This is referred to in traditional acupuncture literature as the Teh Ch'i or Deqi phenomenon.[17] The intensity of cramp parallels that of the severity of muscle shortening: it can be excruciatingly painful, but gradually resolves as shortening eases.

The distribution of the sensation may also be widespread; for example, a needle inserted into the erector spinae muscle at L1–2 may cause Deqi to be felt in the entire length of the muscle, in the low back at the iliac crest, in the gluteal muscles, in the muscles of the abdominal wall, and intra-abdominally. Deqi may be felt on the contralateral side as well.

Release can be hastened by manual agitation of the needle (especially by rapid twisting). As the needle is twisted, both cramp and grasp are intensified, then, typically, both resolve within minutes. Instead of twisting the needle, electrical stimulation with a low-intensity, alternating or interrupted direct current such as is used in transcutaneous electrical nerve stimulation (TENS) may be used.[9,23]

Ordinarily, when several of the most painful shortened muscles in a region have been treated, pain is alleviated in that region. Relaxation and relief in one region often spreads to the entire segment, to the opposite side, and to paraspinal muscles. These observations suggest that needling has produced more than local changes—a reflex neural mechanism involving spinal modulatory system mechanisms, opioid or non-opioid,[6,7] may have been activated. For example, in elbow pain of radiculopathic origin,[18] cervical spinal range is also restricted from paraspinal muscle shortening. When muscles at the elbow are treated, reflex stimulation can extend to paraspinal muscles, and neck range can likewise improve. Localized conditions such as tennis elbow may require only one or two treatments.

RESPONSE IN LONG-STANDING DISORDERS

In conditions of recent onset, when painful points are not numerous, a few treatments separated by days may resolve the pain. But in long-standing disorders, e.g. chronic low back pain, there are many shortened muscles and, more often than not, they include much fibrotic tissue. These fibrotic muscles do not respond as well as normal muscle to needle stimulation. Response is less dramatic and parallels the extent of fibrosis. Since all gradations of fibrotic conversion can exist, the outcome of treatment can vary from individual to individual, from muscle to muscle, and even from one part of the muscle to another. Fibrotic muscle necessitates more frequent and extensive needling; release is limited to individual bands treated, and all tender bands require attention. Treatment of chronic fibrotic conditions, therefore, represents many more needle insertions per session, or more sessions with the same number of penetrations. Several sessions (also separated by days) are customarily needed.[16] When fibrosis is extreme, the needle-grasp is not elicited, even when the needle is vigorously twisted. This indicates that fibrosis has most likely displaced virtually all striated muscle tissue, that contracture is not the cause of pain, and that this method of treatment is not likely to help. The extent of fibrosis does not necessarily equate with chronological age: many older individuals have less wear and tear than younger ones whose musculature has undergone repeated physical or emotional stress[35] or surgery.

FIBROSITIS AND FIBROMYALGIA

The term "fibromyalgia" was coined in 1976 to replace "fibrositis". It describes a soft tissue disorder in which young adults aged 25–50 "hurt all over", complaining of widespread muscle and joint pain, poor sleep, morning stiffness, fatigue and specific "tender points" above and below the waist. In addition, some patients report numbness, cold extremities, weakness, "restless legs", abdominal upsets or menstrual irregularities. There may be stress-linked symptoms such as irritable bowel syndrome, headaches and TMJ. It affects about 3% of the general population, afflicting twice as many women as men. Many sufferers feel too weak to work and incur large compensation costs.

The disorder may be precipitated by some distressing event such as whiplash injury, divorce, bereavement or other emotional experience. Because X-rays and routine laboratory tests yield no underlying organic abnormalities, sufferers are often told that there is "nothing wrong". In 1990, the America College of Rheumatology (ACR) recommended diagnostic criteria that require:

- Diagnosis must exclude other diseases.
- Pain in at least 11 of 18 tender point sites on digital pressure, evaluated by pressing with the thumb or first two or three fingers at a pressure of approximately

4 kg, preferably using a dolorimeter to quantify the pain.

- Pain all over, present for at least three months, on the right and left sides of the body, above and below the waist, with accompanying skeletal pain in the neck (cervical spine) and low back (lumbar spine).
- Poor capacity for muscular exertion (owing to musculoskeletal pain).
- Sleep disturbances—non-refreshing sleep—with frequent night awakenings, diminished REM (rapid eye movement) sleep, possible reduction in alpha sleep waves.
- Brief morning stiffness.
- Intolerance of cold, damp weather.

Much confusion surrounds fibromyalgia and doctors are divided in their opinion about its cause and management. Because fibromyalgia may develop following trauma, or mental distress, some regard it as a physical problem while others consider it as a psychosomatic illness in which problems—such as anxiety, depression, frustration or failure to achieve goals—express themselves.

- Although EEG often shows brain wave patterns with "alpha intrusion in non-REM sleep", fibromyalgia is no longer considered as a sleep disorder.
- Some suggest the disorder arises from abnormal pain sensitivity, possibly caused by abnormal levels of substance P, neurotransmitters, or serotonin.
- There is no consistent link to psychiatric illnesses.

Management

The ACR 1990 criteria have brought despair to countless individuals. Many patients who suffer from widespread musculoskeletal pain are treated as "fibromyalgia", and when their pain fails to respond to popular fibromyalgia treatment (such as tricyclic medications), they are abandoned, as the condition is commonly viewed as a lifetime disorder.

Far from being a distinct syndrome, fibromyalgia merely describes the most extreme and extensive of the mundane aches, pains, and tender muscles that we all have, in various degrees, at one time or other. Mildly tender points are not unusual in asymptomatic individuals, especially after strenuous physical activity, and moderately tender points are not exceptional in those who have a history of a "vulnerable" spine (see Appendix 2). These individuals, although asymptomatic, character-istically have minor degenerative changes visible on roentgenograms. Patients with myofascial pain invariably have multiple tender points; even in localized conditions, such as lateral epicondylitis, examination will reveal numerous tender sites scattered throughout the body—to practised fingers, the number of tender sites in a fibro-myalgic patient can be many times the stipulated number. I prefer the term *"diffuse myofascial pain syndrome"* that has been recommended by The International Association for the Study of Pain (IASP).

Most therapists who have experience of the spine and radiculo-pathy believe that fibromyalgia arises as referred pain from the spine and that the underlying spinal problems need correction to achieve relief. Fibromyalgia's many features— such as widespread aching, point tenderness, skin fold tenderness, articular pain, swelling of the hands or knees, numbness or coldness of the extremities, reticular skin discoloration, irritable bowel and trophedema —indicate a neuropathic origin; these symptoms are manifestations, or epiphenomena, of radiculopathy.

Patients with widespread myofascial pain should unfailingly be given a competent and comprehensive examination of the musculoskeletal system. The examination is never complete without evaluation of the deep paraspinal muscles, especially the intrinsic muscles of the back (e.g. the semispinalis and multifidus muscles).

Treatment starts with reassurance that the condition is not crippling, does not weaken joints or muscles, is not life-threatening and need not hinder a return to work. Place emphasis on muscle conditioning— gradually increasing aerobic exercises such as walking and swimming to upgrade fitness, stretch tight muscles and maintain motion of the joints. Medications such as muscle relaxants may give marginal relief. Antidepressants may relieve the sleep disturbance and alleviate depression.

IMS is an effective technique for examination and specific treatment of fibromyalgia. However, treatment requires needle exploration and treatment of muscles over a wide area in the trunk and limbs. Some commonly tender areas are:

- In the cervical spine and occiput. Examine the suboccipital muscles. It is important to sweep long hair out of the way to reveal any muscle shortening and prominence of the trapezius and semispinalis capitis muscles. With the neck forward flexed, palpate and needle these muscles, aiming the needle at the occiput.

- The longissimus capitis insert into the posterior margin of the mastoid process often requires needling (p. 55).
- The lateral vertebral muscles—the scalenus anterior, medius and posterior are often very tender.
- The trapezius (almost always) and levator scapulae (p. 56).
- The supraspinatus at the musculotendinous junction is frequently tender (p. 63).
- The deep muscles of the spine— the semispinalis, multifidus, and rotatores—are probably the most important and most frequently neglected muscles because they are almost always beyond the reach of palpation and can only be assessed by using a dry-needling technique. These muscles are particularly important in the neck and in the mid-dorsal back (pp. 80–82).
- Lateral epicondyle: common extensor origin and extensor digitorum (p. 67).
- Gluteus medius and piriformis— this deep muscle often requires needling to determine if it is shortened (pp. 88–89).
- Tensor fasciae latae (p. 89).
- Medial knee: the pes anserinus (foot of the goose) is formed by the sartorius, gracilis, and semi-membranosus and semitendinosus (p. 95).
- Tibialis anterior (p. 97).
- Soleus, tibialis posterior (p. 99).

MUSCLE SHORTENING IN PARASPINAL MUSCLES MUST BE TREATED

Treatment, when limited to painful peripheral muscles, can fail if the pain is perpetuated by shortening in paraspinal muscles (at the same segmental levels) that compresses the nerve root.

Prolonged shortening in paraspinal muscles generally defies reflex stimulation and necessitates definitive treatment to decompress the nerve root and thereby break the vicious circle. Traction or manipulation are commonly tried methods, but they often disappoint. In such cases, we have found that accurate and repeated needling of the paraspinal muscles can effectively lead to their release.

In intractable pain of radiculopathic origin, tender bands in myotomal muscles supplied by *both* anterior and posterior primary rami require attention. For example, crepitus and pain may develop in the patella and knee, but tender palpable bands can be demonstrated in the quadriceps femoris muscles, as well as in the paraspinal muscles at the same segmental levels (i.e. at L2–L4).

Paraspinal muscles must be individually palpated for contracture and, if necessary, deeper muscles examined by needling. Each painful constituent muscle (e.g. the semispinalis thoracis) can be identified and treated.

Even when symptoms appear localized to one level, the entire spine needs examination. For instance, back pain is most common at LS–S1 levels, but more often than not, higher segmental levels, frequently reaching dorsal and cervical levels (especially D4, 8, 10, and L2) are involved. After L5–S1, L2 is the second most frequently affected spinal level.

- At involved dermatomes, the skin is often cooler, and trophedema may also be found.
- *Palpation with the palm.* Shortening in paraspinal muscles can be found by palpation with the palm, using the thenar and hypothenar eminences. With the patient prone, *palpate for spinous processes that are more prominent. If tender, needle the paraspinal muscles on both sides of the process, about one centimeter from the midline.*
- Shortening in paraspinal muscles is also confirmed by needle exploration. When paraspinal muscles at consecutive segmental levels are needled, *resistance to needle penetration is substantially increased at the involved level(s)* as compared to the levels above and below.
- **"The invisible lesion." Occasionally, the needle encounters a shortened muscle that seems bony-hard and cannot be penetrated to the depth reached at other levels. Penetration then is only possible by applying some considerable force, and after repeated "pecking".** When the needle finally enters the dense contracture, the patient experiences the intense cramp described above. This gradually diminishes as the needle-grasp is liberated (see p. 35).

Treating chronic pain

The treatment of chronic pain depends on its nature. A source of nociception must be eliminated, inflammation may need rest to permit healing, and anti-inflammatory drugs may be indicated. In neuropathic pain associated with muscle shortening, the release of the shortening usually provides relief. Ordinarily, analgesics or simple physical therapies such as heat or massage, or perhaps more effective measures such as stretching and cooling with ethyl chloride sprays or TENS,[41] may suffice. But in stubborn pain when simple methods prove ineffective, IMS techniques are indicated.

REFLEX STIMULATION

It may be argued that all physical and counterirritational therapies including acupuncture[7] achieve their effect by reflex stimulation since they are effective only if the nerve to the painful part is still intact and partially functioning (a neuropathic nerve is still capable of impulse transmission). Their application excites receptors (in skin and muscle) and stimulates their target indirectly, i.e. by a reflex mechanism. Thus, massage and focal pressure activate tactile and pressure receptors; exercise, traction, and manipulation stimulate muscle spindles and Golgi organs; heat (including ultrasound) and cold act upon thermal receptors. These different stimuli are sensed by their specific receptors and relayed to the spinal cord. As with the patellar reflex, stimulation reaches the affected part indirectly. It is the reflex response in efferent fibers to the affected structure which stimulates the therapeutic target.

Rotation of a needle grasped by muscle shortening can produce intense stimulation. Rotational motion is converted to linear motion which shortens the muscle (similar to tightening a clothesline by twisting its mid-portion) and activates muscle spindles and Golgi tendon organs. Unlike other external forms of physical stimulation which are short-lived, i.e. their stimulation ceases when application is discontinued, needling can provide long-lasting stimulation from the injury it creates. Injury potentials of several micro-amperes are generated and can persist and provide stimulation for days until the miniature wounds heal.[11,13,22] Such stimulation can reach deep muscles (especially paraspinal muscles) which are otherwise not accessible.

Pain in tendons and joints caused by mechanical pull is eased when the shortened muscles acting upon them are released. Improvement can be demonstrated by an increase in joint range; also, minor degrees of joint effusion may resolve. These changes can occur within minutes.

Autonomic dysfunction also responds to needle stimulation: relaxation of smooth muscle can spread to the entire segment, releasing vasospasm (increasing skin temperature) and lympho-constriction.[9,23]

We have studied the efficacy of dry needling in a randomized clinical trial for intractable low back pain.[16] The study could not be double-blind for technical reasons. Progress was assessed by examination for signs of neuropathy, and by return to gainful employment. A long-term follow-up (average 27.3 weeks) showed that the treated group fared significantly better than the control group.

CONCLUSION

Chronic musculoskeletal pain represents a far greater problem than is generally recognized. When chronic pain persists in the absence of detectable injury or inflammation, radiculopathy must be suspected. In radiculopathic pain, muscle shortening is a crucial ingredient: it can cause pain in muscles, tendons, their connective tissue attachments, and joints. Treatment demands the release of muscle shortening. Commonly used physical therapies are usually ineffective, and a needle technique is nearly always necessary.

REFERENCES FOR PART I

1. Asbury A K, Fields H L 1984 Pain due to peripheral nerve damage: an hypothesis. Neurology 34: 1587–1590
2. Bonica J J 1953 The management of pain. Lea and Febiger, Philadelphia
3. Bonica J J 1979 Causalgia and other reflex sympathetic dystrophies. In: Bonica J J, Liebeskind J C, Albe-Fessard D G (eds) Advances in pain research and therapy, vol 3. Raven Press, New York, pp 141–166
4. Bradley W G 1974 Disorders of peripheral nerves. Blackwell Scientific Publications, Oxford
5. Calliet R 1977 Soft tissue pain and disability. F A Davis, Philadelphia
6. Chapman C R, Benedetti C, Colpitts Y, Gerlach R 1983 Naloxone fails to reverse pain thresholds elevated by acupuncture: acupuncture analgesia reconsidered. Pain 16: 16–29
7. Chiang C Y, Chang C T, Chu H L, Yang L F 1973 Peripheral afferent pathway for acupuncture analgesia. Scientica Sinica 16: 210–217
8. Culp W J, Ochoa J 1982 Abnormal nerves and muscles as impulse generators. Oxford University Press, New York
9. Ernest M, Lee M H M 1985 Sympathetic vasomotor changes induced by manual and electrical acupuncture of the Hoku Point visualized by thermography. Pain 21: 25–34
10. Fields H L 1987 Pain. McGraw-Hill, New York
11. Galvani A 1953 Commentary on electricity. Translated by Robert Montraville Green. Elizabeth Licht, Cambridge
12. Gaw A C, Chang L W, Shaw L C 1975 Efficacy of acupuncture on osteoarthritic pain. New England Journal of Medicine 293: 375–378
13. Gunn C C 1978 Transcutaneous neural stimulation, acupuncture and the current of injury. American Journal of Acupuncture 6: 3; 191–196
14. Gunn C C, Milbrandt W E 1976 Tenderness at motor points—a diagnostic and prognostic aid for low back injury. Journal of Bone and Joint Surgery 6: 815–825
15. Gunn C C, Milbrandt W E 1978 Early and subtle signs in low back sprain. Spine 3: 267–281
16. Gunn C C, Milbrandt W E 1980 Dry needling of muscle motor points for chronic low-back pain; a randomized clinical trial with long-term follow-up. Spine 5: 3; 279–291
17. Gunn C C 1977 The neurological mechanism of needle-grasp in acupuncture. American Journal of Acupuncture 5: 2; 115–120
18. Gunn C C, Milbrandt W E 1976 Tennis elbow and the cervical spine. Canadian Medical Association Journal 114: 803–809
19. Gunn C C, Milbrandt W E 1976 Acupuncture loci: a proposal for their classification according to their relationship to known neural structures. American Journal of Chinese Medicine 4: 183–195
20. Howe J F, Loeser J D, Calvin W H 1977 Mechanosensitivity of dorsal root ganglia and chronically injured axons: a physiological basis for the radicular pain of nerve root compression. Pain 3: 24–41

21. Hubbard D R, Berkoff M 1993 Myofascial trigger points show spontaneous needle EMG activity. Spine 13: 1888

22. Jaffe L F 1985 Extracellular current measurements with a vibrating probe. Trends in Neurosciences 517–521

23. Kaada B 1982 Vasodilatation induced by transcutaneous nerve stimulation in peripheral ischemia (Raynaud's phenomenon and diabetic polyneuropathy). European Heart Journal 3: 303–314

24. Kelley W N, Harris E D, Ruddy S, Sledge C B (eds) 1981 Textbook of rheumatology. Saunders, Philadelphia, pp 3–7, 83–96

25. Kirkaldy-Willis W H, Wedge J H, Yong-Hing K, Reilly J 1978 Pathology and pathogenesis of lumbar spondylosis and stenosis. Spine 3: 319–328

26. Klein L, Dawson M H, Heiple K G 1977 Turnover of collagen in the adult rat after denervation. Journal of Bone and Joint Surgery 59A: 1065–1067

27. Lewit K 1979 The needle effect in the relief of myofascial pain. Pain 6: 83–90

28. Loh L, Nathan P W 1978 Painful peripheral states and sympathetic blocks. Journal of Neurology Neurosurgery and Psychiatry 41: 664–671

29. McCain G 1983 Fibromyositis. Clinical Review 38: 197–207

30. Melzack R, Stillwell D M, Fox E J 1977 Acupuncture points for pain: correlations and implications. Pain 3: 3–23

31. Noordenbos W 1979 Sensory findings in painful trauma nerve lesions. In: Bonica J J, Liebeskind J C, Albe-Fessard D G (eds) Advances in pain research and therapy, vol 3. Raven Press, New York, pp 91–101

32. Ochoa J L, Torebjork E, Marchettini P, Sivak M 1985 Mechanisms of neuropathic pain: cumulative observations, new experiments, and further speculation. In: Fields H L, Dubner R, Cervero F (eds) Advances in pain research and therapy, vol 9. Raven Press, New York

33. Simons D G, Travell J 1981 Letter to editor re: myofascial trigger points, a possible explanation. Pain 10: 106–109

34. Sheon R P, Moskowitz R W, Goldberg V M 1982 Soft tissue rheumatic pain: recognition, management, prevention. Lea and Febiger, Philadelphia

35. Sola A E 1984 Treatment of myofascial pain syndromes. In: Benedetti C, Chapman C R, Morrica G (eds) Advances in pain research and therapy, vol. 7. Raven Press, New York, pp 467–485

36. Sola A E 1981 Myofascial trigger point therapy. Resident and Staff Physician 27: 8; 38–46

37. Staub N C, Taylor A E 1984 Edema. Raven Press, New York, pp 273–275, 463–486, 657–675

38. Thomas P K 1984 Symptomatology and differential diagnosis of peripheral neuropathy: clinical features and differential diagnosis. In: Dyck P J, Thomas P K, Lambert E H, Bunge R (eds) Peripheral neuropathy, vol II. W B Saunders, Philadelphia, pp 1169–1190

39. Tichauer E R 1977 The objective corroboration of back pain through thermography. Journal of Occupational Medicine 19: 727–731

40. Torebjork H E, Ochoa J L, McCann F V 1979 Paresthesiae: abnormal impulse generation in sensory nerves in man. Acta Physiologica Scandinavica 105: 518–520

41. Travell J, Simons D G 1983 Myofascial pain and dysfunction: the trigger point manual. Williams and Wilkins, Baltimore

42. Upton A R M, McComas A J 1973 The double crush in nerve entrapment syndromes. Lancet 18: 359–362

43. Wall P D 1979 On the relation of injury to pain, the John J. Bonica Lecture. Pain 6: 253–264

44. Wall P D 1979 Changes in damaged nerve and their sensory consequences. In: Bonica J J, Liebeskind J C, Albe-Fessard D G (eds) Advances in pain research and therapy, vol 3. Raven Press, New York, pp 39–50

45. Wall P D, Devor J 1978 Physiology of sensation after peripheral nerve injury, regeneration, and neuroma formation. In: Waxman S G (ed) Physiology and pathobiology of axons. Raven Press, New York, pp 377–388

46. Wilkinson J 1971 Cervical spondylosis: its early diagnosis and treatment. W B Saunders, Philadelphia

47. Zimmerman M 1979 Peripheral and central nervous mechanisms of nociception, pain, and pain therapy: facts and hypotheses. In: Bonica J J, Liebeskind J C, Albe-Fessard D G (eds) Advances in pain research and therapy, vol 3. Raven Press, New York, pp 3–37

Part 2

Intramuscular stimulation in practice

Summary

Chronic* pain may be due to:

1. **Ongoing nociception**.
   To treat: find and remove source of nociception.

2. *Or* **ongoing inflammation**. Look for signs of inflammation. If none, investigate for abnormal immunologic response.
   To treat: rest, analgesics, anti-inflammatory drugs.

3. *Or* **radiculopathic pain**. Caused by abnormal sensitivity in receptors or abnormal pathways in peripheral nerves. The most common cause is spondylosis, therefore look for signs of spondylosis and radiculopathy, especially muscle shortening.

Muscle shortening can:

- compress intramuscular nociceptors
- mechanically stress tendons, their sheaths and attachments, ligaments, bursae, and joints
- compress a disc space, injuring the nerve root and causing radiculopathy
- create a self-perpetuating circle
- lead to fibrosis and contractures.

There is no pain without muscle shortening. To treat:

- Relax muscle shortening and contractures, especially in paraspinal muscles.
- Desensitize by reflex-stimulation with physical therapies. IMS is the most effective method.

---

*non-psychologic

Guidelines for diagnosis

FEATURES OF IMS-TREATABLE PAIN

Musculoskeletal pain of radiculopathic origin has several unusual features:

- **Neuropathy is a diagnostic necessity**
The presence of neuropathy must first be established. Look for signs of spondylosis and neuropathy (radiculopathy), as spondylosis is the most common cause of neuropathy.

- **Unremarkable history**
Spondylotic radiculopathy generally follows a gradual relapsing and remitting course which is silent unless pain is precipitated by an incident which is often so minor that it may pass unnoticed by the patient. The history, therefore, often gives little assistance: pain can arise spontaneously with no history of trauma, or the degree of reported pain far exceeds that of the injury.

- **No signs of denervation**
Unlike spondylotic pain produced by acute trauma, or by a rapidly expanding space-occupying lesion, there are usually no signs of outright denervation (e.g. loss of reflexes). A "routine examination" will therefore yield "negative findings".

- **Secondary pain prominent**
Frequently, it is not primary pain in muscle that predominates, but pain caused by mechanical strain in tendons, ligaments, and joints secondary to muscle shortening.

- **Localized conditions are rare**
Although most musculoskeletal pain syndromes may appear localized to one structure, e.g. "tendonitis" or "tenosynovitis", examination will reveal signs of neuropathy, especially tenderness and shortening in that tendon's muscle as well as in other muscles belonging to the same myotomes. Often, signs can be found affecting that entire side of the body and, to a lesser extent, the contralateral side.

- **Laboratory, radiological and other tests are generally unhelpful**
Diagnosis is primarily by clinical examination with emphasis on palpation to demonstrate the presence of neuropathic dysfunction. Neuropathic dysfunction presents as mixed sensorimotor and autonomic disturbances: these are usually segmental. (There are 31 pairs of spinal nerves, each consisting of motor, sensory, and autonomic fibers.)

MANIFESTATIONS OF NEUROPATHY

Sensory

- **Hyperpathia** in skin: e.g. when the point of a pin is drawn across skin, it is felt more sharply over affected dermatomes.
- **Allodynia**: muscles can be tender, especially over motor points.

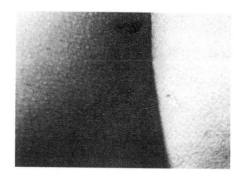

Pilomotor reflex (A).

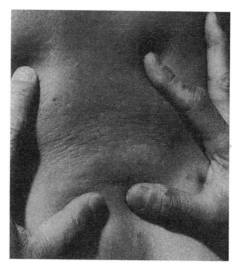

Trophedema (B).

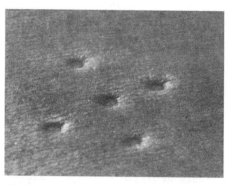

Matchstick test.

Autonomic

- **Vasoconstriction**: affected parts are perceptibly colder.
- **Sudomotor activity**: excessive sweating may follow painful movements or occur after needle treatment.
- **Pilomotor reflex** is often hyperactive and visible as "goose-bumps" in affected dermatomes (A). The reflex can be augmented by pressing upon a tender motor point, especially the upper trapezius.
- **Trophedema** (B), commonly called "cellulite" by the layperson, can be found over affected regions by "skin rolling", that is, by squeezing an area of skin and subcutaneous tissue. In trophedema, the skin is tight and wrinkles absent; subcutaneous tissue consistency is firmer; and the peau d'orange effect and the Matchstick test may be positive.
- **Trophic changes** may occur in skin and nails, and there may be dermatomal hair loss.

Motor

Because pain is primarily related to muscle, signs in muscle are the most relevant and consistent:

- **Muscle shortening**: this key sign may be palpated as ropey bands in muscle which are, in long-standing conditions, sometimes fibrotic (contractures). Focal areas of tenderness and pain in contractures are often referred to as "trigger points". Tender points are usually in the proximity of the painful area, but, in radiculopathy, they can be found throughout the myotome, contralaterally, and in paraspinal muscles.
- **Limitation of joint range** may result from muscle shortening.

- **Enthesopathy**: tendinous attachments to bone are often thickened. Look for enthesopathy at:
  - —insertion of semispinalis capitis at the occiput
  - —longissimus capitis at the mastoid process
  - —deltoid insertion
  - —common extensor origin at lateral epicondyle of elbow
  - —origin of erector spinae.

IDENTIFICATION OF INVOLVED SEGMENTS

In **radiculopathy**, signs are found in the affected segment, in its dermatome, myotome, and sclerotome and in the territories of both anterior and posterior primary rami. Generally, signs are symmetrical: even when symptoms are unilateral, there are latent signs on the contralateral side.

Signs of radiculopathy, especially in muscles, identify the levels of segmental involvement (see Table II). For example, pain may be felt in the knee and patella, but tenderness and painful bands in the quadriceps femoris muscles implicate L2–L4. When painful bands are also found in muscles supplied by the posterior primary rami (the erector spinae muscles) at the same segmental levels, the nerve root is involved.

The entire spine must be examined. The paraspinal muscles should not be summarily dismissed as a collective group. Each individual constituent muscle (e.g. the iliocostalis lumborum) can be palpated and treated if necessary. Furthermore, because many paraspinal muscles such as the longissimus extend throughout most of the length of the spine, the entire spine is examined even when

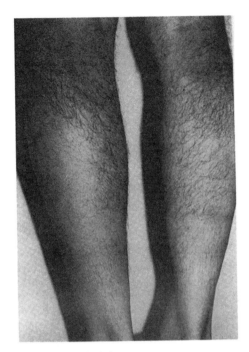

Dermatomal hair loss.

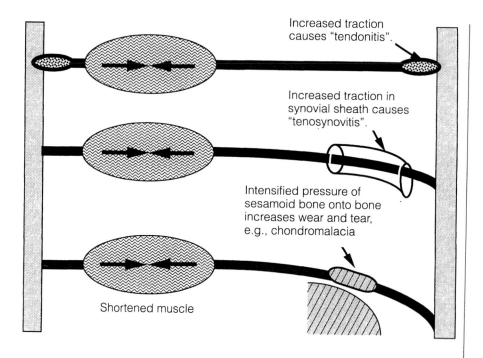

Increased traction causes "tendonitis".

Increased traction in synovial sheath causes "tenosynovitis".

Intensified pressure of sesamoid bone onto bone increases wear and tear, e.g., chondromalacia

Shortened muscle

symptoms are localized to one region. For example, low back pain is most common at L5–S1; but, more often than not, higher segmental levels are involved, frequently reaching dorsal levels. **Contracture in deep muscles can only be demonstrated by needle exploration.**

Specific effects

Muscle shortening can produce pain in a variety of ways:

- Muscle shortening can produce primary muscle pain, and its release eases the pressure in intramuscular nociceptors.
- Muscle shortening mechanically stresses tendons, increasing wear and tear. "Tenosynovitis", "tendonitis", or "trigger finger" can occur.
- If a sesamoid bone is in the tendon, there can be abrasion and pain, e.g. "chondromalacia patellae".
- Increased traction at the muscle origin and/or insertion can cause pain (e.g. "lateral epicondylitis"). When the muscle and/or tendon is long, the pain can manifest some distance away. For example:
  —The *flexor digitorum longus* muscle can produce pain in the sole.
  —The *flexor digitorum profundus* muscle can produce pain at the bases of distal phalanges.
  —The *erector spinae (longissimus)* muscle can produce headache or pain in the neck.
  —The *gluteus maximus* and *tensor fasciae latae* muscles can pull upon the iliotibial tract and cause pain at the lateral aspect of the knee (lateral condyle of tibia).

- Pressure over a bursa can cause "bursitis".
- Altered alignment and restricted joint range due to muscle shortening can cause pain, degenerative changes, and deformity in the joint, as in osteoarthritis and "hallux valgus".
- Muscle pressure upon a nerve can produce an entrapment syndrome: for example, spasm in the *pronator teres* or *pronator quadratus* can compress the median nerve and give rise to symptoms of a carpal tunnel syndrome.
- Shortening of paraspinal muscles across a disc space can perpetuate neuropathy. Increased pressure can eventually lead to disc degeneration and a prolapsed disc.
- Spondylolisthesis.

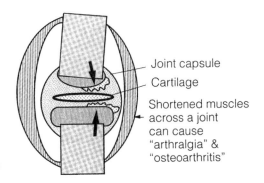

Joint capsule

Cartilage

Shortened muscles across a joint can cause "arthralgia" & "osteoarthritis"

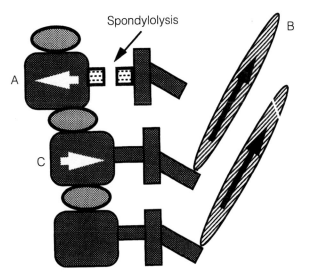

Spondylolisthesis is usually described as a vertebra with spondylolysis sliding anteriorly on the vertebra below (A). However, it is the strong intrinsic back muscles that have shortened (B) and pulled the lower vertebra posteriorly (C).

Treatment and needle technique

Considerations

IMS treatment presupposes that other causes of pain (for example, neoplastic, rheumatoid, etc.) have been eliminated or defined.

IMS cannot reverse structural defects such as advanced changes in osteoarthritis, bony encroachment into spinal nerve foramina, or a torn anterior cruciate ligament in the knee. Response to treatment is also generally unsatisfactory following surgery when there is extensive scarring.

A brief therapeutic trial may be elected on pragmatic grounds. For example, headaches and backaches are extremely common, but extensive investigations are not always indicated. When there are signs of neuropathy, especially muscle shortening and tenderness (see Guidelines for diagnosis), the condition may be amenable to dry needling: if so, there should be a favorable response following a few treatments.

Treatment goals

The primary objective is not to produce analgesia, but to desensitize supersensitive structures and restore motion and function.

● *Release muscle shortening*. This improves the range of joint motion. Muscle shortening is an inherent ingredient of musculoskeletal pain and its release forms the primary part of treatment.

● *Remove the source of irritation at the spine*. Localized pain (e.g. tennis elbow) may often be relieved by needling muscles close to the painful part. But when persistent pain is caused by radiculopathy, nerve irritation at the spine caused by shortened paraspinal muscles that compress the nerve root must also be treated.

● *Promote healing*. Needling produces local inflammation which is the necessary prelude to healing; growth factors, such as the platelet-derived growth factor, are also released. Since both subjective and objective improvement in chronic conditions proceed gradually, a healing process is involved. The

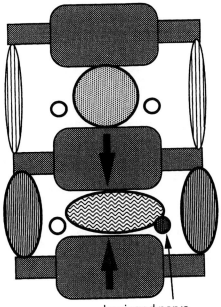

Impinged nerve

condition may be considered as reversed when both symptoms and signs are eliminated and do not recur.

Treatment in anxiety states— "stresspoints"

Anxiety nearly always accompanies pain: body tone is frequently increased, and groups of muscles become tensed and shortened in a characteristic pattern. In chronic pain with anxiety, even when symptoms are localized to one region, many latent points of tenderness, usually symmetrical, may be found throughout the body, i.e. "fibromyalgia" or "diffuse myofascial pain syndrome". These conditions cannot be satisfactorily treated unless anxiety is also controlled. In anxiety, all tender "stress" muscles (those that are called into action in "fight or flight" or protection situations) require treatment.

Some important stress muscles are:

- trapezius
- sternocleidomastoid
- masseter
- prime extensors of the vertebral column

- infraspinatus
- gluteus maximus and medius
- adductor magnus and longus
- pectineus.

Release of stress

Treatment of these muscles, especially the trapezius, can lead to a state of general somatic relaxation (see Dorsal back). Anxiety may be allayed, and medications can usually be discontinued. Following treatment of these "stress" points, patients may experience a feeling of emotional unshackling that they find difficult to describe. Patients may break into unbridled tears of relief, crying without check for many minutes, sometimes up to an hour.

In some chronic pain conditions, e.g. headache, low back pain, "fibrositis", and temporomandibular joint pain, there can be a strong psychosomatic component. Such conditions can not respond to treatment unless the "stress" muscles (especially the trapezius and adductors) are also treated.

NEEDLE TECHNIQUE

Choice of needles

We use stainless steel acupuncture needles: these are finer than hypodermic needles, and their pointed tips minimize trauma to nerves and other tissues. The fine needle allows multiple, closely spaced insertions (sometimes only a few millimeters apart) into individual muscle fasciculi.

The whippy nature of the fine needle transmits the character of penetrated tissues (e.g. fibrous tissue) to the therapist: the procedure is

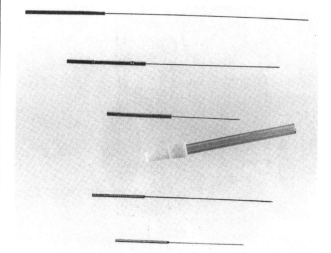

therefore also diagnostic, locating spasm and fibrous contractures in deep muscles where they are otherwise undetectable.

Fine needles (30 gauge or finer) are selected for most muscles; but for thick and strong muscles, such as the gluteus maximus, the preferred minimum diameter is at least 30 gauge: any finer needle would be bent by muscle contraction. The length of the needle (½, 1, 2, 2½, and 3 inches) is also chosen according to the muscle being treated: a thicker muscle requires a longer needle. Early conditions can respond to superficial stimulation using a short and fine needle, e.g. ½ to 1 inch, and multiple insertions; chronic condi- tions with extensive muscle fibrosis require deep and closely spaced penetration with a longer needle.

Finding points

The most effective sites for the release of spasm are situated at the muscle's zone of innervation which lies deep under the motor point, and at musculotendinous junctions. Musculotendinous junctions are easily located by palpation: they are usually tender and often thickened (enthesopathy). The locations of motor points are generally less well known; these (many muscles have more than one motor point) are illustrated in the manual. The exact location of a motor point of a muscle may vary slightly from patient to patient, but the relative position follows a fairly fixed pattern. Some zones of innervation are superficial and are easily found, but those belonging to deep muscles are more difficult to locate with the needle. Piercing a muscle generates an electrical discharge (known to electromyographers as "insertion activity") which is strongly exaggerated in neuropathy: some- times, when the needle accurately enters the zone of innervation, the discharge may cause the muscle to fasciculate and relax.

Using a point-finder or neurometer
In recent years, the dermometer, now renamed the neurometer, has been adopted for point location. The neurometer is a simple instrument powered by dry cells (generally 9–21 V) and consists of a milli- ammeter with a probe and ground or

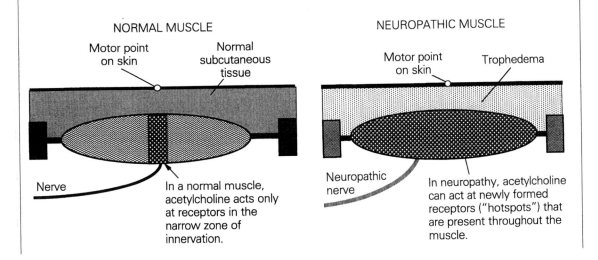

NORMAL MUSCLE

Motor point on skin

Normal subcutaneous tissue

Nerve

In a normal muscle, acetylcholine acts only at receptors in the narrow zone of innervation.

NEUROPATHIC MUSCLE

Motor point on skin

Trophedema

Neuropathic nerve

In neuropathy, acetylcholine can act at newly formed receptors ("hotspots") that are present throughout the muscle.

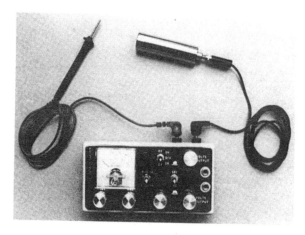

Needle insertion

The direction of needle insertion is generally perpendicular to the skin. To facilitate penetration and to avoid handling the needle, a tubular guide may be used. Nothing or a brief, sharp prick may be felt when the needle penetrates skin. Therefore the needle is given a swift tap to penetrate skin. This is important as it minimizes the sharp pain of penetration, especially in hyperpathic conditions.

When many bands require treatment, several needles may be deployed. A number, e.g. eight, are inserted into tender muscles. When spasm is released in these muscles some minutes later, the needles are withdrawn and reinserted into another selection of muscles.

The use of only one needle, held in a plunger-type needle holder, is recommended as it is most convenient when many muscles require treatment. The plunger-type needle holder allows great accuracy and control in muscle needling. Accurate penetration releases spasm more quickly, and the same needle can be employed sequentially at multiple loci. With the plunger-type needle holder, the speedy release of muscle shortening permits the outcome of needling to be assessed as treatment proceeds.

indifferent electrode. The indifferent electrode is held in the hand of the patient while the probe explores the body surface for areas where resistance to direct current is lowest. When the probe alights on such a point, it emits an audible signal and the milliammeter shows a higher reading.

The neurometer is not specific; it indicates a skin point that has low electrical resistance (e.g. over a zone of innervation), but not all such points are necessarily motor points. In practice, a neurometer is not always necessary because muscle bands that require attention are, as a rule, palpable and tender, and thus easily found.

Finding contractures

When needling, check for the needle-grasp which confirms muscle contracture. When the needle enters a muscle band that is shortened, there is increased resistance to penetration. The needle is then grasped by the shortened muscle—the contraction may be so intense that the needle cannot be easily withdrawn. Simul-

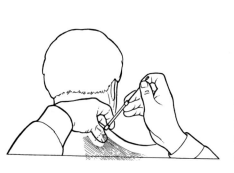

taneously, the patient experiences a cramp-like sensation which can be exquisitely painful. If the patient cannot tolerate the pain, it may be minimized by slowly insinuating the needle, millimeter by millimeter, into the contracture.

The patient's communication of the cramp is the best guide to accurate needling. If spasm is not encountered at the initial insertion, the needle should be partially withdrawn leaving its tip within skin. The angle and depth of penetration should be slightly changed, and the needle pushed in again. The needle-grasp can also often be induced by twisting the needle. The absence of the needle-grasp signifies that the condition is unlikely to respond to this type of treatment.

Release of muscle shortening

Shortening may be released by simply leaving the grasped needle in situ for typically 10–20 minutes. Manual stimulation by "twirling" or "pecking" movements can cause the muscle shortening to initially intensify and then relax more quickly. Although placing the needle at the motor zone or at the musculotendinous junction is most effective in neuropathy, extrajunctional acetylcholine receptors or "hot spots" are formed throughout the entire length of the muscle (see p. 33). Thus a needle inserted almost anywhere into a shortened muscle can release it. Objective release of shortening usually leads to subjective pain relief.

Electrical stimulation

Muscle shortening may also be released by electrical stimulation. Electrical stimulation with a neuro-

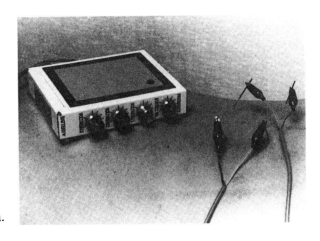

meter point-finder may be applied in the form of a low-voltage (9–18 V) interrupted direct current administered for seconds or minutes to the inserted needle until release is obtained. The frequency and pulse width of the stimulating current are not critical, but a low frequency (see next paragraph) with sufficient current input can cause the muscle to contract. It is often expeditious to combine needling with electrical stimulation. The probe is held in contact with the exposed end of the needle as it is embedded and explores muscle tissue. When the needle contacts an excitable muscle zone, the muscle will contract. Contractions in neuropathic muscle are more easily induced, and are more vigorous than in normal muscle.

Electrical stimulation may also be applied for approximately 15–30 minutes through pairs of TENS (transcutaneous electrical nerve stimulation) electrode leads attached with alligator clips to needles inserted into motor points. The current is gradually increased until muscle contractions are visible: these confirm that the needles are properly placed. Release of contractures occurs best when the stimulation frequency allows the muscle to relax between contractions and not summate to produce tetanic contraction. The summation frequency (about 30–100 Hz) varies from muscle to muscle, e.g. that of the soleus muscle at about 30 Hz is much lower than that of the tibialis anterior muscle at about 100 Hz.

A hand-held point-finder is also useful to relax contracture. See page 122.

Low level laser therapy (LLLT)

Low level laser therapy (LLLT) uses low energy lasers in order to achieve therapeutic effects. Conventional light is a mixture of all colors emitting in all directions. Laser light is monochromatic, coherent, and polarized. Infra red laser light is suitable for deeper lesions. LLLT is safe to use: photo-energy emission is low and treatment is painless, aseptic, and non-thermal. There are no known significant side-effects. There has been no report of eye injury from low level laser, although care must be taken not to stare into the probe. Light from LLLT lasers does not induce cancer growth.

LLLT has anti-inflammatory and analgesic properties; it accelerates the wound healing process. LLLT is useful in myofascial pain and works well for conditions such as epicondylitis, TMJ dysfunction, pain in the neck, herpes simplex, herpes zoster and post-zoster neuralgia, rotator cuff syndrome (frozen shoulder), carpal tunnel syndrome, acute and low back pain, sprain and post-traumatic swelling (hematoma). Laser therapy, with the benefit of painless healing, is widely used instead of needles. Its use complements needle therapy, but its effect is superficial and does not equal that of the needle.*

Treatment of fibrotic contractures

When fibrosis has become a feature of muscle shortening (i.e. contractures), response to treatment is less rewarding. Treatment of extensively fibrotic contractures necessitates more frequent and extensive needling. Release is limited only to individual muscle bands treated: to relieve pain in such a muscle, all tender bands require needling. This implies more needle insertions per session, or more sessions with the same number of insertions.

Multiple needle insertions, sometimes as closely spaced as a few millimeters apart, may be necessary to release a muscle band. The pointed, "atraumatic" needle produces minimal trauma, but occasionally small blood vessels may be pierced, and the patient should be warned that there may be some soft tissue swelling and bruising. Occasionally, a bulge may appear at the site of insertion. Digital pressure applied for a few minutes, or low level laser therapy (LLLT) electrical stimulation will relax this. When all palpably tender bands have been needled, allodynia and joint range should improve within minutes.

Patients should be told that there may be minor discomfort and some bruising from the needling for a day or two, and that the pain may occasionally become worse before it improves.

---

*Pontinen P J 1992 Low level laser therapy as a medical treatment modality. Art Urpo, Tampere.

CAUTIONS

Contraindications

IMS is a safe procedure in the hands of physicians who have a knowledge of anatomy. There are few contraindications:

- early pregnancy
- local infection
- hemophilia (or patient is on anticoagulants).

Precautions

IMS needles are disposable, or sterilized by autoclaving. Whereas the author follows standard precautionary non-touch techniques for asepsis (hands scrubbed with no gloves, as these impair the sense of touch for accurate palpation), each therapist must make a personal choice regarding the use of gloves—a choice made more difficult by the risk of the transmission of HIV/ARC/AIDS. The possibility of infection cannot be excluded in any population. In needling and palpation, the therapist will likely come in direct contact with the patient's blood or other body fluids. With or without gloves, handling needles always poses the possibility of skin puncture to the therapist. The use of gloves limits tactile sensitivity and makes fine palpation difficult. Whether or not gloves are worn or other precautions taken, it is recommended that the therapist be immunized for hepatitis B.

Mishaps

Accidental penetration of vital structures has been reported in traditional acupuncture literature, but our system is intended for qualified medical personnel. With a knowledge of anatomy, vital organs, large vessels, and nerves can be avoided. When needling, accidental penetration of vital structures can be avoided by carefully identifying landmarks, and palpating each muscle before needle insertion. The depth of penetration into a muscle is dictated by its anatomy. Brief descriptions of relevant muscles are given in this manual, but regular reference to an atlas of anatomy is recommended. Be especially careful when needling the upper trapezius.

On the very rare occasion, an older needle may break off at its hilt. Therefore, penetration should not utilize the full length of the needle; a short protruding length should be left for withdrawal with a pair of forceps. However, with disposable needles, breakage is very unlikely.

Vasovagal reaction

The needling of very tender and sensitive points (especially in the upper trapezius) may induce a pronounced vasovagal reaction. This is likely in tense or nervous individuals (and more commonly in those with fair skin, blue eyes, and blond or reddish hair). The patient quickly recovers when placed in a supine position, with the feet raised. Treatment should be conducted with the patient lying horizontally until, after several treatments, tolerance to needling is established.

General examination

A general examination must always precede the regional examination of the painful part. Examine the entire musculoskeletal system because pain in one location can cause associated muscle shortening in distal parts of the body, particularly on the same side. (Examples: temporomandibular joint pain, "whiplash" neck pain, trigeminal neuralgia—these are always part of a generalized muscular disorder, see under Fibromyalgia.)

Examination should:

• *Establish the presence of neuropathy*. See Guidelines for diagnosis.

• *Determine the affected segments*. Since spondylotic radiculopathy is by far the commonest cause of neuropathic pain, a quick, overall survey to detect segmental dysfunction (most easily discerned in muscles) is described below. With practice, the survey takes but a few minutes. Many physical signs are obvious and are determined simply by observing the patient for discomfort or distress, mood, attitude, stance, gait, general movement, and sitting position.

• *Demonstrate the muscles involved*. Carefully examine the affected region: muscles, tendons, ligaments, connective tissue attachments, and joints. (See Regional examination and specific treatment.)

General assessment

The following short and, with practice, quickly-done general examination of the musculoskeletal system supplements, but does not replace, a regular medical examination, even though the latter may reveal no significant findings.

The patient should be completely undressed and no gown provided, although underpants/brassiere may be retained until the examination requires their removal.

Careful palpation is essential. Any abnormality discovered by the survey directs attention to the affected region.

The general assessment should include examination of the patient in erect, supine, and prone positions. The following format provides a logical progression through the necessary examination steps. IMS-treatable problems are followed by the name of the appropriate reference section in Regional examination and specific treatment. Sections can be found by consulting the names shown on the tab strips. Problems that are structural and not IMS-treatable are marked "Not IMS".

PATIENT ERECT

A full-length mirror is useful for simultaneous observation of the front and back of the patient. The patient faces the mirror, with the examiner standing behind. Look for any obvious muscle wasting and weakness, deformities, skin rashes (e.g. herpes zoster) or discoloration (e.g. peripheral cyanosis, erythema ab igne), or dermatomal hair loss.

Whenever range of motion is limited in a joint, the muscles acting on that joint must be examined by palpation.

Examination of the patient should include the following:

Stance and posture
Some patients stand with a "**chin-up, head forward**" posture. This posture is associated with: (1) a chin that is thrust forward because there is hyperextension at C2–3 or C3–4. (If the extended neck were corrected, the patient would be facing downwards, looking at his feet.) (2) The hyper-extension is necessitated by increased kyphosis in the dorsal spine, plus (3) slight flexion in the hips. The hips cannot be fully extended. The Fabere sign shows restriction, especially of extension, abduction and external rotation in the hips (see below, under Hips). The patient therefore stands and walks with slightly flexed hips. This slight flexion, in addition to slightly increased dorsal kyphosis, causes the patient to be facing downwards; the head is therefore hyperextended in order to correct the abnormal posture.

The "chin-up, head forward" posture is very common. The primary lesion is in the lumbar back at L2 level which causes shortening in the psoas major, pectineus, and hip adductors. The paraspinal muscles at L1, 2, and 3, the adductors, pectineus, sartorius, and sometimes the rectus femoris muscles require treatment before relaxation can be achieved in the neck. Next to L5–S1, L1–2 or L2–3 are the most commonly injured levels.

Gait
- Limping?
  Continue assessment.

Standing on heels
If this is not possible:
- Is the problem in the ankle joint (structural)?
  Not IMS.
- Is dorsiflexion (tibialis anterior) weak?
  See Leg.
- Is extension of the big toe (extensor hallucis longus) weak?
  See Leg.
- Are calf muscles shortened?
  See Calf.

Standing on toes
Not possible?
- Is the problem in the foot/ankle joint?
  Not IMS.
- Is tibialis anterior shortened?
  See Leg.
- Are calf muscles weak?
  See Calf.

Full squat
Not possible?
- Check hip joints.
  See Buttock.
- Check knee joint.
  See Thigh.
- Are quadriceps shortened?
  See Thigh.
- Check low back.
  See Back.

Is the pelvis level?
No? Measure leg lengths.
- Discrepancies of ½" or less don't usually require shoe lifts.
  See Leg.
- Uneven leg lengths? (Discrepancies greater than ½".)
  Not IMS.
- Problem in hip and knee joints.
  Not IMS.

Trendelenburg's sign

When the patient stands on one leg, the pelvis should rise slightly on the other side, provided that the supporting hip joint is normal and the gluteal muscles on the supporting leg can contract normally.

- Positive? Rare: congenital dislocation of the hip; coxa vara; fracture of the neck of femur; osteochondritis deformans juvenilis.
  Not IMS.
- Weak elevation or false positive? Common: weak gluteal muscles especially gluteus medius.
  See Dorsal back and Buttock.
- Check gluteal muscles and low back (L5–S1).
  See Dorsal back and Buttock.

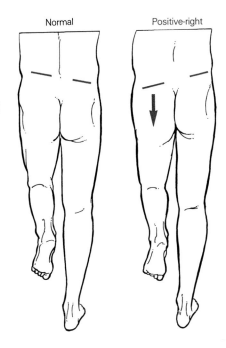

Normal   Positive-right

Spinal curves and range

- Any scoliosis?
  See Lumbar back.
- Increased dorsal kyphosis?
  See Lumbar back.
- Loss of lumbar lordosis?
  See Lumbar back.

Forward flexion

Note that flexion in hips may permit a full range of motion, despite a stiff back.

- When fully flexed, is one side more prominent than the other?
  See Lumbar back.
- Is the tip of any spinous process more prominent? A more prominent spinous process may indicate a level of dysfunction. It is often easier to feel for a slightly raised spinous process by palpating with the palm of the hand, feeling with the thenar or hypothenar pads. Press upon the process—tenderness indicates ongoing pathology.
  See Lumbar back.

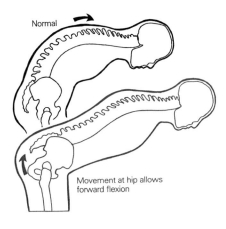

Normal

Movement at hip allows forward flexion

GENERAL EXAMINATION

Extension, lateral rotation, and bending
- Any abnormality? Examine lumbar spine.
  See Lumbar back.

Shoulders
- Is one shoulder higher? If so, is this caused by trapezius/levator scapulae shortening on that side?
  See Shoulder.
- Due to mid-dorsal scoliosis?
  See Shoulder.
- Are both shoulders held too high (chronic anxiety)?
  See Shoulder.
- Examine neck and shoulders.
  See Shoulder.

Glenohumeral range
Fix the scapula with one hand holding the tip of scapula between thumb and index finger, then passively abduct the arm.
- Limited on one side? (N = 70–80 degrees.)
  See Shoulder.
- Examine shoulder.
  See Shoulder.

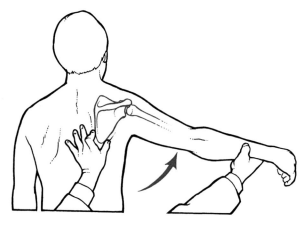

Neck
- Forward flexion: chin should reach chest.
  See Cervical spine.
- Lateral rotation: 60–70 degrees, but when forced, chin should almost reach shoulder.
  See Cervical spine.
- Lateral bending: about 45 degrees.
  See Cervical spine.
- Extension: the examiner's finger is trapped between the occiput and C7 spinous process.
  See Cervical spine.
- Limited? Painful? Examine neck.
  See Cervical spine.

Radial pulses

The combined modified Adson's and costoclavicular maneuver is a test for thoracic outlet syndrome. With the patient seated, take the radial pulse on the affected side. Continue to note the pulse while performing the following:

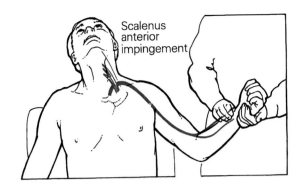

- To test for scalenus anterior impingement, while continuing to take the pulse, have the patient take a deep breath, **hold chin up, extend head**.
- To check for scalenus medius impingement, lift and abduct the arm to a horizontal position and have the patient rotate the head away from the affected side.

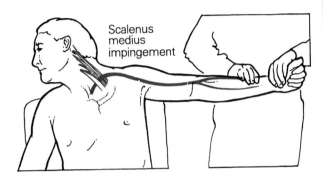

- To see if the neurovascular bundle is compressed by insertion of the pectoralis minor at the coracoid process, hyperabduct and hyper-extend the arm, lifting it above the level of the patient's head.
- Positive (pulse loss occurs)? *See Cervical spine and Shoulder.*

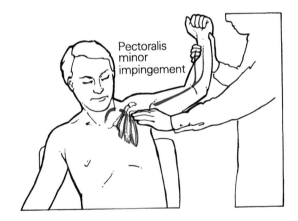

PATIENT SUPINE

Lower extremities

The examination of the lower extremities must always include the lumbar back.

- Any muscle wasting?
- Any tenderness at motor points?
- Any dermatomal hair loss? *See Back.*
- Examine lumbar back. Tenderness in muscles of a myotome indicates the segment involved. *See Back.*
- Straight leg raising: limited? *See Back and Thigh.*
- Lasegue's sign (pain along course of sciatic nerve when it is put to

GENERAL EXAMINATION

stretch by flexing the hip and extending the knee): positive? *See Back and Thigh.*

- Examine low back and hamstrings. *See Back and Thigh.*

Hips

Fabere (F-Ab-ER-E) sign. When the heel of the painful side is placed on the knee of the other leg, the knee on the affected side remains elevated and cannot be depressed; i.e. there is pain on attempted Flexion, Abduction, External Rotation, and Extension.

Patrick's sign is a different test; it resembles the Fabere sign, but in Patrick's the hip is passively moved to determine if there is any loss of range.

- Positive? Limited? Painful? *See Thigh.*
- Check hip joint. *See Buttock.*
- Are adductors shortened? *See Back.*
- Examine the low back (especially L2–L3). *See Back, also see Posture and chin forward position.*

Knees

- Stability: ruptured cruciate/ collateral ligaments? *Not IMS.*
- Effusion? *See Thigh.*
- Range-flexion: limited? Is the problem in the joint? *Not IMS.*
- Quadriceps: wasting? (measure at 10 cm above upper pole of patella); strength; muscles shortened? *See Thigh.*
- Extension: limited? (Quick check: a fully extended knee does not allow the examiner's hand to slide under it.) Limitation of extension is usually caused by shortening in the hamstring, and pes anserinus.

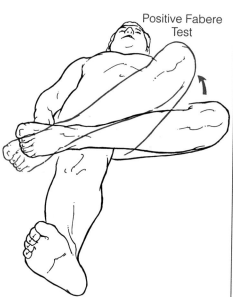

Positive Fabere Test

- Are hamstrings or pes anserinus shortened? *See Thigh.*

Anterior chest and body

- Gently run the point of a pin down the body across dermatomes. Segmental hyperpathia indicates level of dysfunction.
- Clavicles level? A–C joint tender? *See Shoulder.*
- Check pectoralis major, trapezius, and sternomastoid. *See Shoulder.*
- Squeeze anterior/posterior axillary folds: tender? *See Shoulder.*
- Examine shoulder. *See Shoulder.*

Upper extremities

Examination of the upper extremities always includes the cervical spine.

Elbows

- Is extension limited? Is the problem in the joint?
  Not IMS.
- Are biceps, brachioradialis, and brachialis shortened?
  See Elbow.
- Is flexion limited? Is the problem in the joint?
  Not IMS.
- Are triceps shortened?
  See Elbow.

Radioulnar joints

- Is pronation limited? Check supinator and biceps.
  See Elbow.
- Is supination limited? Examine pronators, flexor carpi radialis, anconeus.
  See Elbow.

Wrists

- Flexion limited? Check wrist extensor muscles.
  See Elbow.
- Extension limited? Check wrist flexor muscles.
  See Wrist.

Hands

- Muscle wasting? Trophic changes in nails?
  See Wrist.
- Cold fingers? Peripheral cyanosis?
  See Wrist.
- Tender interossei muscles?
  See Wrist.
- Clawing? Examine wrist flexors.
  See Elbow.
- Dupuytren's contracture? Examine wrist flexors, especially palmaris longus.
  See Wrist.

PATIENT PRONE

Use a thin (about 4″) pillow placed under the abdomen to straighten lumbar lordosis; allow the arms to hang down by the sides of the couch, drawing the scapulae laterally and exposing the posterior thorax.

- Gently run the point of a pin down the body, crossing dermatomes. Segmental hyperpathia indicates the level of dysfunction.
- Check for skin temperature (significant changes are usually perceptible by palpation).
  See Back.

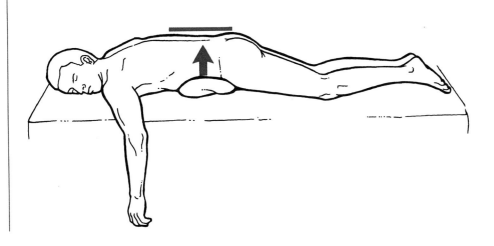

- Trophedema. Skin rolling test.
  See Back.
- Matchstick test positive?
  See Back.
- Examine low back.
  See Back.

Palpate the upper (squeeze between fingers), mid and lower trapezius, posterior deltoid, rhomboids, latissimus dorsi.
- Tender? Examine neck and shoulders.
  See Cervical spine and Shoulder.

Palpate muscles of:
- Back.
  See Back.
- Buttocks.
  See Buttock.

- Palpate with flat of palm for any increased prominence of spinous process; press down to check for tenderness.
  See Back.

Palpate and check for tenderness in:
- Hamstrings.
  See Buttock.
- Calves.
  See Calf.
- Soles.
  See Calf.

Regional examination and specific treatment

The regional examination follows a general examination. The vertebral column usually consists of 33 vertebrae, 24 of which are movable (7 cervical, 12 thoracic, and 5 lumbar). In musculoskeletal disorders of spondylotic (i.e. radiculopathic) origin, pain can arise from any segmental nerve, but for examination and treatment purposes, the body may be divided into the following regions:

1. **Cervical spine**
2. **Upper limb**
   a. **Shoulder**
   b. **Elbow and forearm**
   c. **Wrist and hand**
3. **Back**
   a. **Dorsal back**
   b. **Lumbar back**
4. **Lower limb**
   a. **Buttock and posterior thigh**
   b. **Anterior thigh and knee**
   c. **Leg and dorsum of foot**
   d. **Calf**
   e. **Foot**

These regions, peripheral and spinal, are innervated respectively by the anterior and posterior primary rami of segmental nerves. **Examination of any one part of the body should include both its spinal and peripheral regions**. For example, the upper limb has developed from, and represents a morphologic extension of the cervical spine; thus, the examination of an elbow (a peripheral region) should also include the neck (its spinal region).

To perform an examination:

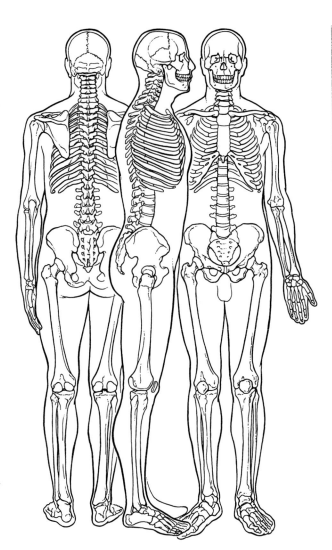

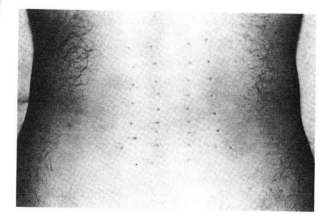

- Note any cutis anserina ("goose-bumps") or hair loss in affected dermatomes.
- Palpate for tender and painful bands in shortened muscles. Usually, the most tender areas of a muscle are at its midportion, where it is most prominent when contracted, and at musculotendinous junctions.
- Check for trophedema with the Matchstick test (see p. 26). Usually, the cutaneous tissues over the most tender muscle bands have the deepest indentations.
- Examine for restricted range of motion (active and passive) in joints activated by the shortened muscles.
- Examine the intrinsic muscles of the back (see Back, pp. 80–82). The intrinsic muscles of the back (which are concerned with maintenance of posture and movements of the vertebral column) span the entire length of the back. These muscles (especially the erector spinae) are almost always found to be shortened and therefore require treatment in spondylotic pain syndromes. These muscles bend the spine laterally, usually to the affected side, and their shortening can increase the pressure on disc spaces at several levels. Because spondylotic changes affect the entire disc space, even when pain presents only on one side, signs of neuropathy including shortened muscles can usually be found on the contralateral side. Treatment should always include both sides.

Note that narrowing of a disc space is usually accompanied by:

- Prominent tip of spinous process which is tender to pressure; and

- Skin crease at the same level. X-rays of the spine will usually reveal some degenerative changes, e.g. narrowing of a cervical disc is accompanied by a skin crease in the neck.

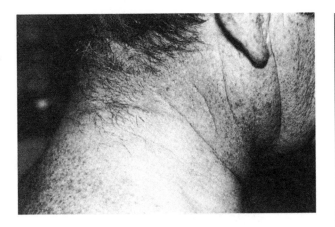

Cervical spine

EXAMINATION

Identify bony landmarks

Find the external occipital protuberance and superior nuchal line.
The spinous process of C2 (axis) is the
first palpable bony point below the
external occipital protuberance. The
next easily palpable spinous process
is C7. Identify transverse processes of
C1 (atlas) which are palpable about
1 inch inferior to the tips of the
mastoid processes. To count the
vertebrae, begin with T1: each
spinous process overlies the body of
the vertebra below it. For example,
the spinous process of C6 overlies the
body of C7.

Trophedema in the suboccipital region

This is an important area where
trophedema often appears. Soft tissue
appears boggy, and the occiput cannot
be palpated. The upper musculotendinous ends of the trapezius and
semispinalis capitis muscles can be
enthesopathic and thickened. When
the head is forward flexed, these
appear very prominent on one or
both sides, and are very tender.

Palpate muscles

Palpate for tender, taut bands of
shortening in muscles. Unless there
is extensive fibrosis, not all muscles
require treatment, as reflex stimulation from treated muscles can spread

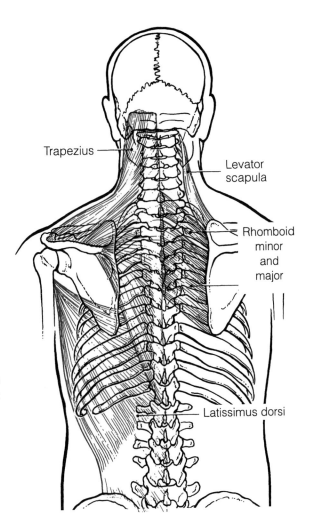

Trapezius

Levator
scapula

Rhomboid
minor
and
major

Latissimus dorsi

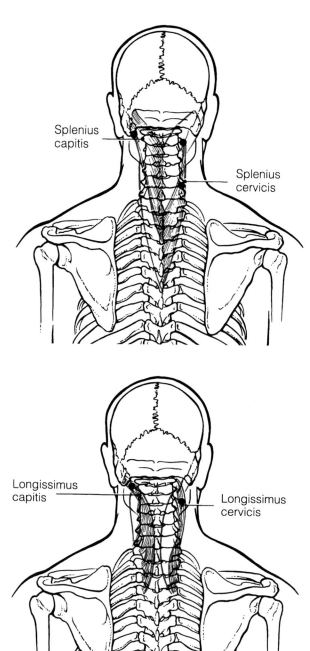

Splenius capitis

Splenius cervicis

Longissimus capitis

Longissimus cervicis

to other muscles within the same segment. There are four layers of posterior cervical muscles; the needle can pierce one or more layers as required:

Layer 1
This includes the superficial extrinsic muscles: the *trapezius, latissimus dorsi, levator scapulae,* and *rhomboids* which connect the upper limb to the axial skeleton. Also see Upper limb.

Layer 2
The intrinsic back muscles include the *splenius capitis* and *cervicis*. (Common origin is from lower half of the ligamentum nuchae and spinous processes of C7–T6. The splenius capitis inserts into the mastoid process, and the splenius cervicis into the transverse processes of the upper two to four cervical vertebrae.)

Layer 3
This layer is formed by the erector spinae muscle. In the neck, it is represented by the *longissimus capitis* and *cervicis* muscles. (These extend from the pelvis: the capitis inserts into the mastoid process, and the cervicis into the posterior tubercles of the transverse processes of C2–C6.)

Layer 4

This is the deep layer of intrinsic back muscles: the *semispinalis capitis* (the transverse processes of the upper thoracic and the articular processes of the lower cervical vertebrae, into the occipital bone between superior and inferior nuchal lines near the midline), the *multifidi*, and *rotatores* (also see Back).

Lateral aspect of neck

This includes the *levator scapulae* (the posterior tubercles of the transverse processes of the upper cervical vertebrae to the vertebral border of the scapula between the superior angle and spine of scapula), *scalenus anterior* (the scalene tubercle of the first rib to the anterior tubercles of the middle cervical vertebrae), *scalenus medius* (the upper surface of the first rib behind the subclavian groove to the posterior tubercles of the middle cervical vertebrae), *scalenus posterior* (the posterior part of the second rib to the posterior tubercles of the lower cervical vertebrae), *sternomastoid* (the medial head from the manubrium sterni, the lateral head from the upper surface of the medial third of the clavicle to the mastoid process and the lateral part of the superior nuchal line).

Check range of neck motion

Stand behind the seated patient and check the range of neck motion:

Forward flexion

The chin should reach the chest. Any limitation is caused by shortening in the *splenius capitis* and *cervicis*, *semispinalis capitis* and *cervicis*, *iliocostalis cervicis*, *longissimus capitis* and *cervicis*, *trapezius*, and *interspinalis* muscles.

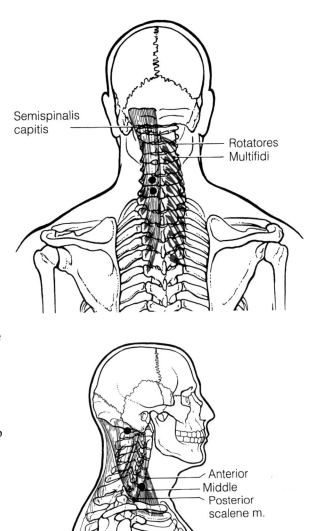

Semispinalis capitis

Rotatores
Multifidi

Anterior
Middle
Posterior
scalene m.

CERVICAL SPINE

Lateral rotation

This should be 60 degrees, but with persuasion the chin should almost reach the anterior shoulder. Any limitation is caused by shortening in the contralateral *splenius capitis* and *cervicis, sternomastoid, scalenes, longissimus capitis, multifidus, levator scapulae* muscles, and the ipsilateral upper trapezius muscle.

Lateral tilting

This should be 45 degrees. Limitation is indicated by palpable shortening in the contralateral muscles, especially the scalenes.

TREATMENT

Treatment of the neck should include treatment to the shoulders and upper limbs. Often, the entire spine has to be treated.

Not infrequently, a tight neck is secondary to the chin-up, head forward posture. Check to see if the neck is hyperextended at C2–3–4, where there will be a deeply recessed spinous process.

Position of patient

Prone, with a shallow pillow to support the chest and allow the neck to flex.

Alternate position

Sitting, with neck flexed and forehead supported on a table. Because of the possibility of a vasovagal reaction, the sitting position should not be used until the patient has had previous treatments and has shown good tolerance to needling.

To improve forward flexion

Treat the *semispinalis capitis* and

cervicis at C5 level. This should improve forward flexion.

If not, continue with the following. Identify the external occipital protuberance, superior nuchal line and transverse processes of C1. Palpate for and treat the attachments of the *trapezius, semispinalis capitis,* and *splenius capitis* muscles with the needle aimed at the occiput. (Sometimes treating the semispinalis can, by itself, improve flexion.)

At the mastoid process, palpate for, and needle the *longissimus capitis* and *sternomastoid* muscles which lie deep to the splenius capitis.

Identify spinous processes C1–C6. **Do not needle immediately medial to the transverse processes of C1 because the vertebral artery lies in the suboccipital triangle**. Palpate and needle the *semispinalis capitis, longissimus capitis,* and *cervicis*

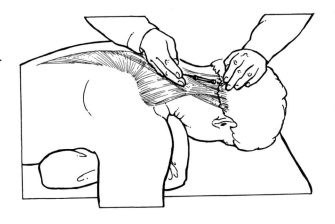

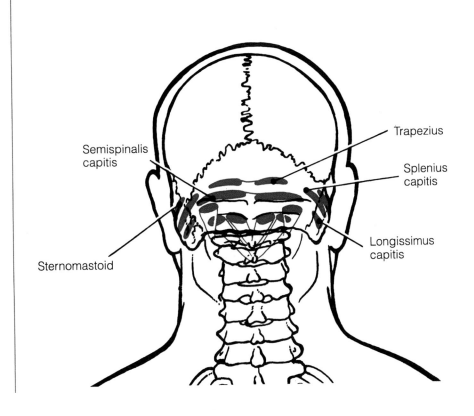

Semispinalis
capitis

Trapezius

Splenius
capitis

Longissimus
capitis

Sternomastoid

Needle trapezius from posterior aspect

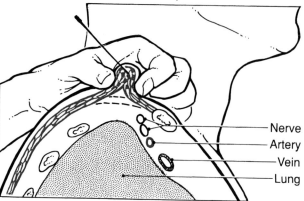

— Nerve
— Artery
— Vein
— Lung

Important: Carefully grip and isolate the trapezius muscles, and needle from posterior aspect to avoid piercing the lung.

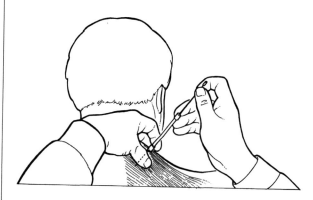

muscles through the *splenius capitis* at about ½, ¾, and 1 inch from the midline at C5 and, if necessary, at C4 and C6. Then reach deeper to treat the multifidi and rotatores muscles.

When paraspinal muscles at consecutive segmental levels are needled, **resistance to needle penetration can be substantially increased at the involved level(s)** as compared to the segmental levels above and below. The needle can encounter spasm that seems bony-hard, and penetration cannot attain the depth reached at other levels. Penetration is only possible after repeated "pecking" and the application of some force. This dense, fibrotic tissue is an important clinical finding as it is not revealed by radiological, CAT, or MRI techniques.

Recheck the range of flexion, which should be improved.

To improve lateral rotation

Lateral rotation is limited by shortening in the ipsilateral upper *trapezius* and the contralateral *splenius capitis* and *cervicis*. Grip the upper edge of the ipsilateral *trapezius* muscle between thumb and index finger. Carefully needle all palpable

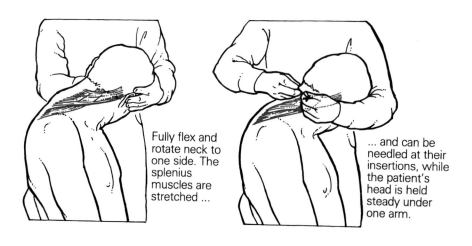

Fully flex and rotate neck to one side. The splenius muscles are stretched ...

... and can be needled at their insertions, while the patient's head is held steady under one arm.

muscle bands from the posterior aspect. Needling of this muscle can occasionally cause a severe vasovagal reaction, often associated with nausea. **Do not insert the needle vertically from the superior aspect, because the apex of the lung lies beneath**. Also needle the trapezius just superior to the spine of the scapula. It is convenient at this stage to treat the supraspinatus muscle (see Shoulder, p. 63).

Check the range of lateral rotation; in most patients it should be improved. If flexion is not improved, fully flex and rotate the neck to the restricted side: the *splenius capitis* and *splenius cervicis* on the other side are then stretched and can be reneedled.

To improve lateral bending

Have the patient recline semiprone with the treatment side up. Tilt the head away from the treatment side. Identify and laterally needle the upper attachments of *levator scapulae*, *scalenus medius*, and *posterior* muscles at the posterior tubercles of the transverse processes of the cervical vertebrae and aim at the tips of the transverse processes. Needle only taut muscles, and avoid the lower part of the posterior triangle formed by the anterior border of *trapezius*, posterior border of *sternomastoid*, and the clavicle.

The sternomastoid muscle is treated next. Instruct the patient to slightly lift the head off the pillow to tense the *sternomastoid* muscle. Needle the upper portion of the muscle about 1 to 2 inches below the mastoid process, avoiding the external jugular vein.

Check the range of lateral flexion, which should be improved. Palpation should, by this stage, reveal a softer

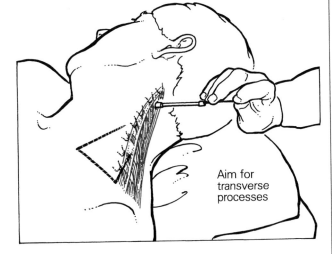

Aim for transverse processes

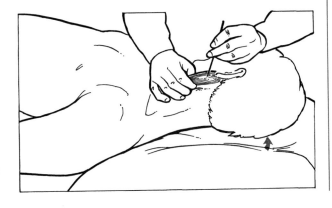

and much more supple neck. Identify and treat residual taut and tender muscle bands.

The "Whiplash" syndrome

This syndrome, more often than not, affects the entire spine. Palpate the entire spine (with patient prone and using the palm of the hand) for prominent and tender spinous processes that indicate the level(s) of injury. All muscles supplied by cervical nerves in the neck and upper limb should be examined and palpated, especially the *trapezius*, *splenius capitis* and *cervicis*, *longissimus capitis* and *cervicis*, and *semispinalis capitis* muscles.

On the painful side, the *levator scapulae* is frequently shortened (see Shoulder, p. 63) and the "Hammer lock" test is positive (see p. 62). Treat the neck as described above.

Check for range of motion. **Forward flexion** is usually limited, especially by shortening of *semi-spinalis capitis*. Measure by using "number of fingerbreadths" between chin and chest. **Lateral rotation** is usually limited by shortening in the ipsilateral upper *trapezius* and the contralateral *splenius capitis* and *cervicis*. If pain is worse on one side of the neck, there is usually a compensatory scoliosis in the dorsal back on the other side to keep the head vertical, and another on the ipsilateral side in the lumbar back. Treat taut sides to realign back to normal. Also examine and treat any tender muscles in the upper limbs, usually the muscles of the shoulder and at the lateral aspect of the elbow. As anxiety is a frequent companion to the syndrome, examine the "stress muscles" (see Treatment in anxiety states).

Also palpate and treat the dorsal spine, if necessary—the *spinalis thoracis* and *semispinalis*. It is often necessary to explore with a needle, inserting it to reach the spine, but **keeping the needle to within one finger's breadth from the midline**. Search especially for tenderness at D6, 8 to D10, and on both sides of any tender, prominent spinous processes.

Palpate and treat, if necessary, the *longissimus*, *iliocostalis*, *multifidi* and *quadratus lumborum* muscles in the lumbar back. The *gluteus medius* is nearly always tender. Check Trendelenberg's test.

Headaches

Almost all headaches are referred from the cervical spine. The three most common types of headache are muscle contraction (or tension) headaches, migraine, and cluster headaches. There is no laboratory or X-ray test that will diagnose these. The diagnosis is suggested by a history that is typical of one of them, and there is usually no need for investigation. Treatment may be started when there are no abnormalities on clinical examination, and its progress can be gauged by observing the response to treatment. However, there are seven danger signals that suggest the possibility of serious disease:

- failure of the headache to conform readily to an innocuous pattern
- onset of headache in childhood or middle age (45–50)
- recent onset and progressive course
- other neurological or general symptoms
- the patient "looks sick" or "isn't right"
- abnormal physical signs
- meningeal irritation.

Muscle contraction headache is believed to be caused by sustained tension of the scalp and neck muscles. It is extremely common and usually reflects a tense or depressed emotional state precipitated or aggravated by stress or fatigue. It may also occur from eyestrain, e.g. working for prolonged periods at a desk or staring into a computer terminal. Pain is usually diffuse, bilateral, and often described as tight or pressing. In most people, tension headaches last for hours or a few days. Constant tension headaches lasting weeks or months usually signal an underlying depression.

Physical examination is normal, save for the finding of tender and shortened muscles in the neck and shoulders. These muscles can be tender during and sometimes between headaches. Trauma may injure neck muscles and cause neck pain and headache. The majority of muscle contraction headaches are believed to have an emotional component.

Migraine is produced by dilatation and increased pulsation of the arteries of the scalp and face. It affects women oftener than men. Attacks may be triggered by stress and fatigue, menstruation and ovulation, alcohol, chocolate, cheese, and other foods. The classic migraine can be associated with aura, visual distortions, confusion, or dysphasia. IMS reduces the number of treatments necessary and some patients have not had migraines for weeks after treatment.

Cluster headache is also vascular in origin, but differs from migraine in its predilection for males in the third to fifth decade. Cluster headaches cluster in time. They occur one or more times a day, every day, for weeks or months, and then disappear completely, only to return months or

years later. Each headache is the same. It begins abruptly, often in the small hours of the morning. The pain is excruciating. It centers around one eye (always the same eye in any cluster) and may spread into the cheek, temple, or forehead. There is redness, a partial or total Horner's syndrome, and running of the ipsilateral nostril. The pain lasts some 20–90 minutes, and then clears—only to return again.

Tic douloureux (trigeminal neuralgia) is a disease of the elderly, characterized by severe unilateral facial pain lasting a second or two at most. It is triggered by touching certain parts of the face, and severe, recurrent lancinations can pierce the cheek, gum, or jaw.

All three types of headaches are associated with muscle contraction in the neck and they generally all respond well to IMS treatment of the cervical spine when the restricted range of motion in the neck is restored. In tic douloureux, the *splenius capitis* and *cervicis*, suboccipital muscles, *masseter* and *levator labii superioris* are also treated.

The difficult headache

The severity and frequency of all types of headaches can be diminished by IMS. Frontal headache responds to needling of suboccipital muscles. Temporal headache and ringing in the ears (tinnitus) respond to needling of the upper *trapezius* and *splenius capitis* and *cervicis* muscles. **However, in some patients, the headache persists unless tender points scattered over the entire body are treated.**

Temporomandibular joint dysfunction

This common condition is part of a

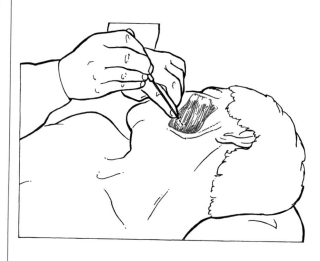

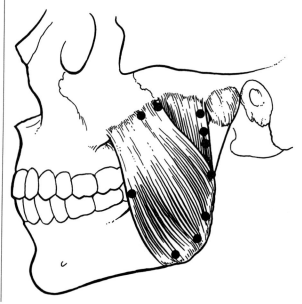

generalized musculoskeletal pain disorder, typically associated with anxiety and stress. **All "stress muscles" must be examined and treated if necessary**. (TMJ is often treated by dentists with night splints—these help, but there is rarely necessity for major dental procedures such as changing the bite, lengthening the teeth or caps. TMJ is not fundamentally a dental condition.)

Treatment is to the jaw and neck, especially the *upper trapezius, splenius capitis* and *cervicis, scalenes* and *paraspinal* muscles. But before treating the jaw, measure mouth opening by the number of fingers that can be inserted between incisors.

Ask the patient to clench the teeth. Palpate for and needle, with a fine 1-inch needle, all bands of muscle shortening in the masseter (these are small and closely spaced). (The masseter stretches from the inferior margin and deep surface of the zygomatic arch to the lateral surface of the ramus and coronoid process of the mandible.) With a fine needle, the parotid gland may be penetrated without hazard.

Needle the bands close to their origin at the zygoma; there is usually a thick and dense band, just anterior to the joint, that inserts into the coronoid process.

Ask the patient to fully open the mouth; the important anterior bands are stretched and needled.

Next, needle the bands as they insert into the ramus. Re-palpate the muscle, which should be softer; the mouth should open wider. Needle any residual taut bands. (It is rarely necessary to treat the pterygoids. These may be identified with a finger in the open mouth. They are needled through the masseter.)

Upper limb

Shoulder

EXAMINATION

Identify bony landmarks

Anterior aspect: clavicle, acromion, humerus (lesser tuberosity, inter-tubercular groove), coracoid process, acromioclavicular joint.

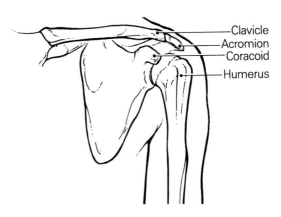

Posterior aspect: the spinous process of T1, scapula (superior and inferior angles at levels of T2 and T7 spinous processes), medial and lateral borders of scapula, spine of scapula; humerus (greater tubercle, surgical neck, and deltoid tuberosity).

Pain in the shoulder can be due to shortening in:

- the muscles connecting the upper limb to the vertebral column
- the muscles that pass from the scapula to the humerus and act on the shoulder joint.

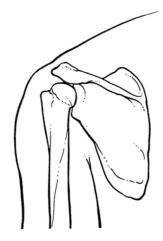

Palpate muscles

Palpate the muscles for tender points and spasm. Examination should include:

- Muscles connecting the upper limb to the vertebral column: trapezius, latissimus dorsi, levator scapulae, and the minor and major rhomboids.
- Muscles that pass from the scapula to the humerus and act on the shoulder joint: deltoid, teres major, supraspinatus, infraspinatus, teres minor, and subscapularis.

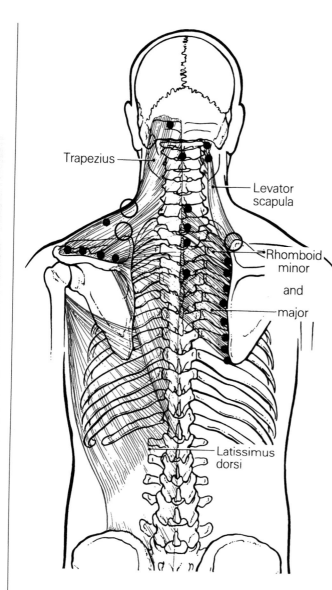

Superficial

Trapezius: the medial third of the superior nuchal line, external occipital protuberance, ligamentum nuchae, and spinous processes of C7–T12 to the lateral third of clavicle, acromion, spine of scapula, and base of scapular spine.

Latissimus dorsi: from the spines of the lower six thoracic vertebrae, lumbar fascia, outer lip of iliac crest, lower three or four ribs, and by an occasional slip from the inferior angle of the scapula to the bottom of the bicipital groove of the humerus in front of the teres major. As it turns around the lower border of the teres major, it forms the posterior fold of the axilla.

Deep

Levator scapulae: from the posterior tubercles of the transverse processes of the upper cervical vertebrae to the medial border of the scapula between the superior angle and spine of the scapula.

Rhomboid minor: from the ligamentum nuchae and spine of C7 to the medial border of the scapula opposite the spine of the scapula.

Rhomboid major: from the spines of the upper five thoracic vertebrae to the vertebral border of the scapula below the rhomboid minor.

"Hammer lock" test

Shortening in the trapezius, levator scapulae, and rhomboids pulls the scapula superiorly and medially, so that the superior angle of the scapula can be palpated above its normal level at D2.

We have devised the "Hammer lock" test to check for this shortening. With the patient prone, place the arm into full internal rotation posteriorly.

If these muscles are shortened, the elbow is lifted away from the table. You can measure the distance from tip of shoulder to table. It never fails to impress the patient when the elbow returns to normal in one session when the levator scapulae and rhomboids are treated. To treat the levator scapulae, palpate and needle the superior angle of the scapula. To treat the rhomboids, have someone press down on the elbow—this lifts the medial border of the scapula which can then be needled.

Muscles that pass from the scapula to the humerus and act on the shoulder joint

Deltoid: from the lateral third of the anterior border of the clavicle, lateral edge of acromion, and the whole length of the lower border of the spine of the scapula to the lateral surface of the humerus just above the middle.

Teres major: from the dorsal surface of the scapula at the inferior angle to the medial lip of the bicipital groove of the humerus.

Supraspinatus, infraspinatus, and teres minor muscles: arise from the dorsal surface of the scapula, the first from above the spine, the second from below the spine, and the teres minor from the axillary border. They insert into the greater tuberosity of the humerus.

Subscapularis: from the ventral surface of the scapula to the lesser tuberosity of the humerus (not easily reached).

These last four scapular muscles make up the rotator cuff.

TREATMENT

Treatment of the shoulder always

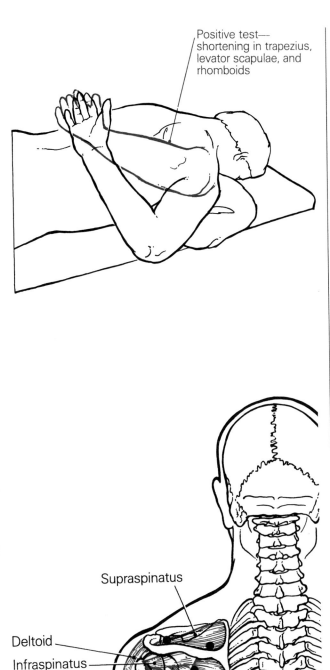

Positive test—shortening in trapezius, levator scapulae, and rhomboids

Supraspinatus
Deltoid
Infraspinatus
Teres minor
Teres major

UPPER LIMB • SHOULDER

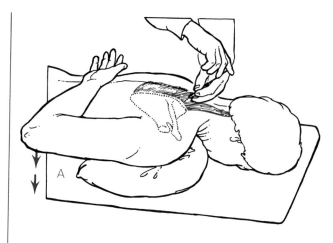

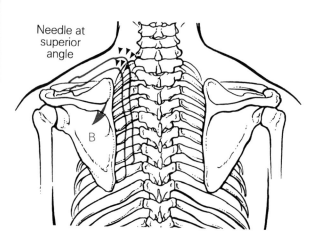

Needle at superior angle

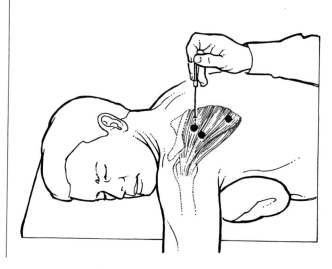

includes the paraspinal muscles of the neck.

Shortening in the trapezius, levator scapulae, and rhomboids

Needle the attachments of these muscles at the superior angle and medial border of the scapula. The elbow gradually lowers as the muscles are needled. With repeated needle insertions, **the elbow can often be returned to its normal position in one treatment session (A).** (Also see Cervical spine.)

The release of muscle shortening can be confirmed by observing puncture marks. With muscle release, the scapula migrates inferiorly and laterally. Although at each insertion the needle is repeatedly directed at the same bony point, the superior angle of the scapula, each succeeding insertion enters the skin at a point that is inferior and lateral to the previous one (B).

A restricted glenohumoral range

Compare one side to the other: normal range is approximately 70–90 degrees. Restricted range is usually caused by shortening of the *infraspinatus, teres minor,* and *latissimus dorsi* muscles. Abduct the arm to 90 degrees to stretch and treat the above muscles.

Pain and restriction on abduction

When there is pain in the first 30 degrees of abduction, treat the rotator cuff muscles: *supraspinatus, infraspinatus,* and *teres minor.* The *supraspinatus* should be treated at its lateral portion where the scapula protects the lung. This muscle is thicker than is generally appreciated and often a 2-inch needle is needed. The sub-scapularis usually relaxes from reflex stimulation when these muscles are treated. If necessary, it can be reached through the posterior axillary fold when the arm is abducted and pulled laterally.

When there is a painful arc from 60–120 degrees

Treat as above, but also treat the deltoid, especially the deep, middle fibers over the surgical neck of the humerus and at the deltoid tuberosity. Use a 2-inch long needle to penetrate the full depth of the muscle and reach underlying bone.

To treat pain and restriction on extension

Extend the arm forward and needle the tight posterior portion of the deltoid, teres major, infraspinatus, and latissimus dorsi.

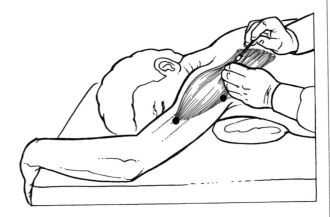

To treat pain and restriction on internal rotation posteriorly

For example, when there is pain and difficulty when putting the thumb between scapulae. Abduct the arm to about 90 degrees. Grasp the anterior axillary fold between thumb and fingers, with fingers tucked well under the fold to protect the axillary vessels and brachial plexus. Needle the lateral portion of the pectoralis major at its musculotendinous junction. (From the medial half of the front of the clavicle, the front of sternum and cartilages of the upper six ribs, and the aponeurosis of the external oblique to the lateral lip of

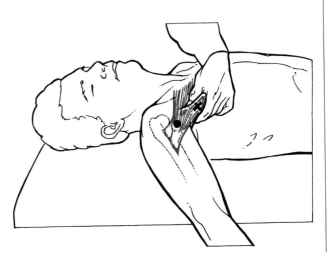

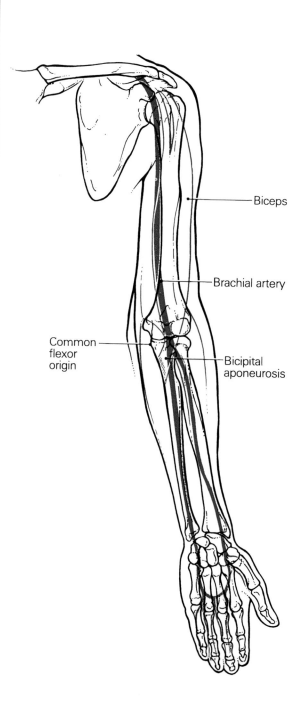

Biceps

Brachial artery

Common flexor origin

Bicipital aponeurosis

the bicipital groove of the humerus. The tendon consists of two layers: the anterior receives clavicular and upper sternal fibers; the posterior gives attachment to lower thoracic fibers which ascend deep to the upper part.)

When the pectoralis major is relaxed, with the arm abducted, palpate for and carefully needle the *pectoralis minor* muscle at the coracoid process through the pectoralis major.

Also palpate and needle the *tight anterior portion of the deltoid* and, through the deltoid, the long and short heads of the biceps.

The frozen shoulder

The "frozen shoulder" is not restrained by "capsulitis"; all movements are restricted because of muscle shortening. All the above muscles require treatment, especially:

- to increase abduction—treat *infraspinatus, teres minor* and *major*.
- to increase forward elevation—all the above muscles, and also the *subscapularis*.
- to improve internal rotation posteriorly—the *pectoralis major* and *minor*, and *anterior deltoid* muscles.

Elbow and forearm

EXAMINATION

Identify bony landmarks

Humerus: greater and lesser tubercles; intertubular groove and tendon of long head of biceps; deltoid tuberosity; medial and lateral epicondyles.

Radius: head of radius, styloid

process, dorsal tubercle.

Ulna: head and olecranon.

Avoid the course of the brachial artery (which is accompanied by the median nerve and two deep brachial veins) from the medial side of the biceps to the cubital fossa where it ends opposite the head of the radius under cover of the bicipital aponeurosis.

Also note the cubital fossa; its boundary on the ulnar side is the pronator teres and, on the radial side, the brachioradialis: note also the floor, brachioradialis, and supinator.

The elbow consists of three joints: humeroulnar (extension and flexion), radioulnar, and radiohumeral (pronation and supination).

Palpate muscles for tender points and spasm

Check the range of elbow extension ("carrying angle" of about 163 degrees) and flexion, as well as wrist extension and flexion.

Pain in the lateral elbow

This is commonly caused by shortening in the extensor muscles on the back of forearm: *brachioradialis, extensor carpi radialis longus, extensor carpi radialis brevis, extensor digitorum, extensor carpi ulnaris, extensor digiti minimi,* and *anconeus.*

The *brachioradialis* and *extensor carpi radialis longus* arise from the lateral supracondylar ridge of the humerus. The brachioradialis is inserted into the base of the styloid process of the radius. The anconeus arises from the posterior surface of the lateral epicondyle of the humerus to the lateral surface of the olecranon.

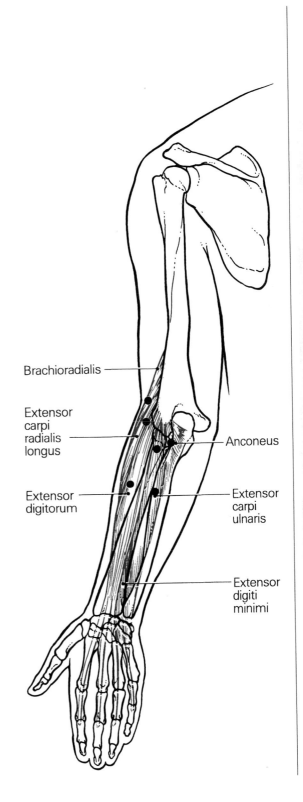

Brachioradialis

Extensor carpi radialis longus

Extensor digitorum

Anconeus

Extensor carpi ulnaris

Extensor digiti minimi

The other four muscles have a common extensor tendon from the front of the lateral epicondyle of the humerus, and also from the deep fascia and from the fibrous septa between adjacent muscles. Insertions of all extensors of the wrist are to the base of the metacarpal bones.

Most of these muscles are easily identified by palpation. With the elbow extended and the palm facing down, the patient is asked to repeatedly extend the fingers or wrist. The activating muscles in the forearm are easily discerned.

Deep to the above muscles are the *supinator, abductor pollicis longus, extensor pollicis brevis, extensor pollicis longus,* and *extensor indicis*. Of these, only the *supinator* may require treatment. To needle the supinator, the forearm must be fully supinated.

Pain in the elbow joint

This can be from:

- Shortening in muscles that flex the forearm at the elbow joint: the *brachialis* (from the anterior surface of the lower half of humerus and intermuscular septa to the front of the coronoid process of the ulna), the *biceps brachii* (long head from the labrum glenoidale, short head from the tip of the coracoid process with the coracobrachialis to the tuberosity of the radius), and the *brachioradialis*.

- Muscles that extend the forearm at the elbow joint: the *triceps brachii* (the long head from the scapula just below the glenoid cavity, lateral and medial heads from the posterior surface of the humeral shaft above and below the spiral groove to the upper surface of the olecranon).

Pain in the medial elbow

This is commonly caused by shortening in the flexor muscles on the front of the forearm: the *pronator teres, flexor carpi radialis, palmaris longus, flexor digitorum sublimis, flexor carpi ulnaris.* The *flexor digitorum sublimis* is the largest and lies at a deeper level. All have a common origin by a tendon from the front of the medial epicondyle of the humerus; the contraction of the common muscle mass on the ulnar side of the elbow is easily felt when flexing wrist or fingers. They also arise from deep fascia and the fibrous septa between adjacent muscles.

Additional heads of origin. Pronator teres, from the humerus above the medial epicondyle and from the coronoid process of the ulna. *Flexor digitorum sublimis,* from the coronoid process and oblique line of the radius. *Flexor carpi ulnaris,* from the medial surface of the olecranon and subcutaneous border of the ulna.

Insertions

Pronator teres, the lateral aspect of the radius about the middle. *Palmaris longus,* the palmar aponeurosis. All flexors of the wrist insert into the base of the metacarpal bones, except the *flexor carpi ulnaris* which inserts into the pisiform bone.

Deep to the above are the *flexor digitorum profundus, flexor pollicis longus,* and *pronator quadratus,* from the anterior surfaces of the radius and ulna.

Anatomical relations

The radial and ulnar arteries run down the forearm on each side, with their accompanying nerves lying nearer the margin: the radial nerve

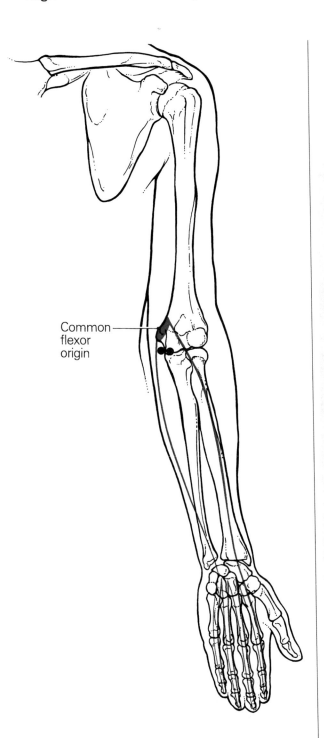

Common flexor origin

reaches the artery from the lateral epicondyle; the ulnar nerve comes from the interval between the olecranon and the medial epicondyle. The median nerve runs distally in the middle of the forearm between the two vessels.

TREATMENT

Treatment of the arm always includes the paraspinal muscles of the neck.

To treat pain and tenderness over the lateral epicondylar region

Pain and tenderness over the lateral epicondylar region upon wrist extension (e.g. "tennis elbow" or lateral epicondylitis) is a common condition that responds well to IMS of the extensor muscles on the back of the forearm: the *brachioradialis*, especially the *extensor carpi radialis longus*, *extensor carpi radialis brevis*, *extensor digitorum*, *extensor carpi ulnaris*, *extensor digiti minimi*, and *anconeus*, but sometimes all tender muscles in the region, for example the *triceps* and *supinator*, must be needled. To access the *supinator* muscle, the arm must be in a supinated position.

1. Degeneration (spondylosis) in the neck causes neuropathy.

2. Neuropathy causes *spasm* and *shortening* of the wrist extensors.

3. Constant pull of wrist extensors on lateral epicondyle causes *Tennis Elbow* and *Tenosynovitis*.

To treat pain and tenderness over the medial epicondylar region

Needle the flexor muscles on the front of the forearm: *pronator teres, flexor carpi radialis, palmaris longus, flexor digitorum sublimis,* and *flexor carpi ulnaris* and their common origin.

Wrist and hand

EXAMINATION

Treatment of the wrist and hand always includes treatment to the cervical spine on both sides.

Pain and dysfunction in the wrist can be due to shortening in:

- The *extensor pollicis longus* and *abductor pollicis brevis* muscles that extend and abduct the thumb. Shortening stresses their tendons and causes friction and tenosynovitis, e.g. **de Quervain's disease.**
- The *pronator quadratus* muscle, causing a deep ache in the distal forearm, between the radius and ulnar bones.
- The muscles that extend and flex the hand at the wrist. This limits wrist extension and/or flexion and causes pain in the forearm and wrist.

TREATMENT

Carpal tunnel syndrome

When the median nerve is trapped within the carpal tunnel (or by shortening in the pronator teres muscle, i.e. "pronator syndrome"), there can

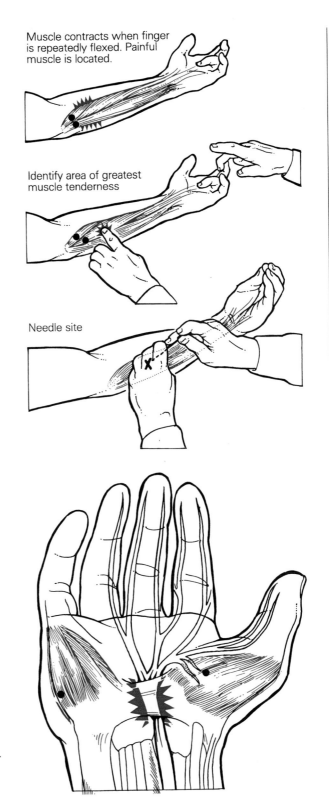

Muscle contracts when finger is repeatedly flexed. Painful muscle is located.

Identify area of greatest muscle tenderness

Needle site

be tingling, numbness, impaired sensation, and pain in the median-nerve-supplied first three fingers and thumb. The symptoms may be reproduced by forced flexion at the wrist, maintained for 2 minutes.

In early cases, before severe muscle wasting occurs in the thenar muscles, the condition responds to needling of the median-supplied muscles in the forearm (*pronator teres* and *quadratus*, and the wrist and finger flexors) and the thenar muscles (*abductor pollicis brevis, opponens pollicis*, and *flexor pollicis brevis*). More often than not, there is "double entrapment" and nerve roots at the cervical spine also require release by needling the paraspinal muscles. In advanced cases, when there has been denervation, results are poor even with surgery.

Trigger fingers

A sudden snapping may occur during flexion and re-extension of a finger or thumb. Palpation usually reveals tender nodules on the flexor tendon within, or proximal to, the synovial sheath. In early cases, the condition responds to treatment of the *flexor digitorum* muscles in the forearm and the direct needling of the nodules and surrounding soft tissues.

Degenerative joint disease

This may occur in relatively young people. The thumb carpometacarpal joint is commonly affected. Pain, tenderness, and stiffness (often bilateral) may impair the grip and fine movements. Early cases respond well to needling of the thenar muscles (*abductor pollicis brevis, opponens pollicis*, and *flexor pollicis brevis*), other muscles acting on the thumb, and especially the dorsal *interossei*.

Pain in the wrist

Treat all muscles that extend and flex, abduct and adduct the hand at the wrist, and the dorsal *interossei*.

Rheumatoid arthritis

This frequently involves the joints of the hand and wrist, affecting the distal and proximal interphalangeal and metacarpophalangeal joints.

For pain in the joints of the fingers: in the forearm, treat muscles that extend (*extensor digitorum, extensor indicis,* and *extensor digiti minimi*) and flex (*flexor digitorum superficialis* and *profundus*) the fingers.

In the hand, needle the dorsal *interossei* muscles with a fine ½ to 1-inch long needle.

With patient's fist clenched, apply firm digital pressure to the muscles between the metacarpals: needle the most tender areas, about 1½ inch proximal to the heads of the meta-carpals where the Matchstick test usually yields the deepest indenta-tion. Angle the insertions medially and laterally to pierce both heads.

In the initial stages, when the disease affects soft tissues and before structural disintegration occurs, relief of pain and swelling can be provided by releasing the shortened muscles that act on these joints. Release relieves stress on tendons and the friction in their sheaths. Treatment repeated at weekly intervals during an acute episode can alleviate the condition and minimize any structural disintegration until the episode has passed. **These comments also apply to rheumatoid arthritis affecting other joints in the body.**

Dupuytren's contracture

Dupuytren's contracture is a painless

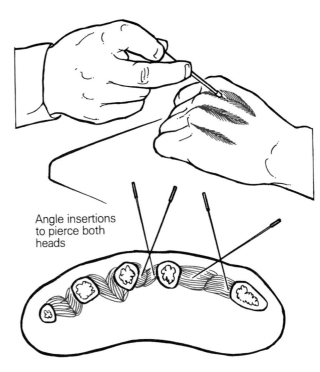

Angle insertions to pierce both heads

condition with fibrosis occurring in the palmar fascia. The fibrosis ultimately progresses to fibrous bands that cause the fingers to contract. Although the flexor tendons are not intrinsically involved, needling their shortened muscles, especially the *palmaris longus* and any nodular lesions in the palmar fascia, can gradually provide worthwhile contracture release in early cases.

Back

Dorsal back

EXAMINATION

Check curvatures of the vertebral column. All thoracic vertebrae articulate with ribs; the spinous processes are long and all are palpable (especially with the palm).

Superficial extrinsic muscles

Examine the muscles as described for Shoulder:

- *trapezius*
- *latissimus dorsi*
- *levator scapulae*
- *rhomboid major*
- *rhomboid minor*.

Spondylotic pain from the dorsal spine

Pain in the dorsal region is generally from shortening of intrinsic back muscles that arise from, or insert into the dorsal spine: the *spinalis*, *semispinalis capitis*, *semispinalis cervicis* and *thoracis*, *multifidus*, and *rotatores*.

Pain may be referred into the lateral and anterior chest wall (intercostal muscles). However, spondylotic symptoms from the dorsal and upper lumbar segments are often visceral via the thoracolumbar sympathetic division of the autonomic system which regulates the internal organs. Symptoms may mimic or even precipitate cardiac

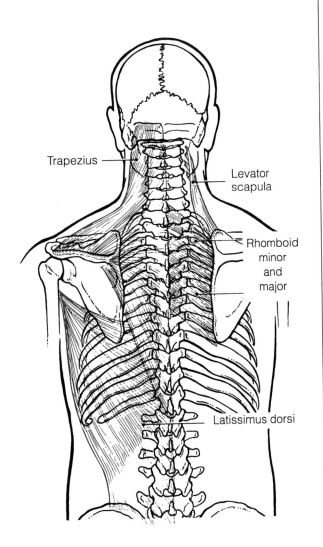

Trapezius

Levator scapula

Rhomboid minor and major

Latissimus dorsi

pain, acute cholecystitis, epigastric pain, irritable bowel syndrome, and dysmenorrhoea (see below and figure of autonomic system).

TREATMENT

The intrinsic back muscles (see Lumbar back) can be needled at segmental levels about ½ inch from the midline. Treatment can also relieve visceral symptoms.

Radiculopathy and segmental autonomic reflexes

The actions of the sympathetic and parasympathetic systems are generally mutually antagonistic. The sympathetic system helps maintain a constant internal body environment, or homeostasis. It commands reactions that protect the individual, such as increase of blood sugar levels, temperature, and regulation of vasomotor tone. The parasympathetic system lacks the unitary character of the sympathetic, and its activity increases in periods of rest and tranquillity. (The traditional Chinese term "Rebalancing the Yin and Yang"—Yin and Yang represent opposing forces—probably emphasizes the necessary balance between the two autonomic systems.)

Sympathetic fibers in spinal nerves innervate the blood vessels of skin and muscle, pilomotor muscles, and sweat glands. In emergency situations, there is a generalized sympathetic discharge, and fibers that are normally silent at rest are activated: sweat glands, pilomotor fibers, adrenal medulla, and vaso-dilator fibers to muscles. In radiculo-pathy, comparable reactions occur in the affected segment **which indeed behaves as if it were in a state of**

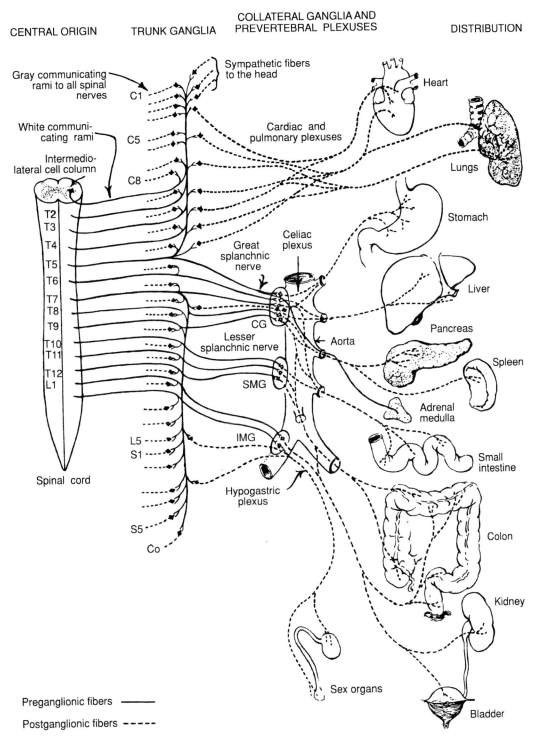

Sympathetic division of the autonomic nervous system (left half). CG—celiac ganglion; SMG—superior mesenteric ganglion; IMG—inferior mesenteric ganglion. (From de Groot and Chusid 1991 Correlative Neuroanatomy, 21st edn. With permission from Appleton and Lange, Norwalk, Connecticut, USA)

B A C K • D O R S A L B A C K

emergency. Vasoconstriction gives radiculopathy its cardinal feature—affected parts are discernibly colder, as may be shown by thermography. The pilomotor reflex is alerted, which may be manifested as "goose-bumps" in the involved dermatome; sudomotor activity may be profuse too.

Sympathetic fibers in visceral nerves innervate the intestine, intestinal blood vessels, heart, kidney, spleen, and other organs (see figure). As with the somatic system, afferent impulses from the viscera connect with motor efferent neurons of the autonomic system in the spinal cord and brain stem. Fibers to the different visceral effectors are independent and discrete, and commands are carried out in reflex fashion. (Early acupuncturists undoubtedly noticed the association between the autonomic system and viscera—thus naming meridians after them.)

Although modulation of autonomic reflexes is carried out in the CNS, supersensitive segmental autonomic reflexes can be influenced and restored to normal by releasing muscle contractures in involved segments. For example, epiphenomena (or manifestations) of radiculopathy, such as tension headache, cluster headache, even migraine, and allergic rhinitis, improve when supersensitive sympathetic nerve fibers are restored to normal.

Upper gastrointestinal (GI) complaints are common, but symptoms like heartburn, gastroesophageal reflux, non-ulcer dyspepsia, and peptic ulcer disease are often difficult to differentiate from those of the *irritable bowel syndrome* (abdominal pain, abdominal distention, relief of pain with defecation, frequent stools with pain onset, loose stools with pain onset, mucus passage, and the

sensation of incomplete evacuation or tenesmus). The two groups of symptoms may indicate, respectively, dysfunction in the greater and the lesser splanchnic nerves.

Upper GI complaints are usually associated with mid-dorsal back pain and signs of spondylotic radiculopathy (such as tenderness and trophedema) in the mid-dorsal back (T2–5). The irritable bowel syndrome is generally associated with the lower dorsal back (T5–L1), but it is not uncommon for a patient to suffer from both groups. Dorsal spondylosis commonly remains silent until symptoms are precipitated by emotional stress or physical strain (lengthy air travel and carrying heavy baggage, for instance).

There is a tendency to over-investigate these symptoms because they can suggest something benign or something serious. Since these symptoms respond quickly to the release of paraspinal muscle contractures in affected segments, however, it is feasible and probably preferable to try IMS first.

Parasympathetic fibers travelling in the vagus nerve are abundant in the thorax and abdomen; they slow the heart, enhance digestion, and produce bronchial constriction. Problems of bronchial constriction and secretion may be relieved with treatment to the cervical and upper dorsal spine.

Lumbar back

EXAMINATION

Check curvatures of the vertebral column

Look for flattening of the normal curvature, lumbar lordosis, scoliosis, and accentuation of scoliosis during flexion.

Check range of motion

Stand behind the erect patient and check the main movements of the vertebral column: forward flexion, extension, lateral bending, and rotation. The range of movement varies according to the individual, but it is important to note if there is any restriction at segmental levels, especially on forward flexion (when distances between spinous processes should be increased).

Identify bony landmarks

The spinous processes of most of the presacral vertebrae can be palpated. Use the palm of the hand to feel for any slight prominence of spinous processes. L2 or 3 is often prominent and tender. If so, do the Fabere test. After L5–S1, L2–3 is the most frequently injured segment. This leads to limitation of extension of hips, and contributes to the "chin-up, head forward" posture (see p. 40). A line joining the skin dimples formed by the posterior superior iliac crests crosses the spinous process of the second sacral vertebra. Palpate the iliac crest and iliolumbar ligament. Palpate the 12th rib, quadratus lumborum, and external oblique muscle.

Palpate for trophedema, and determine where it is most intense by the Matchstick test.

Identify the intrinsic muscles of the back

The intrinsic or true muscles of the back form paired muscle columns on each side of the spinous processes;

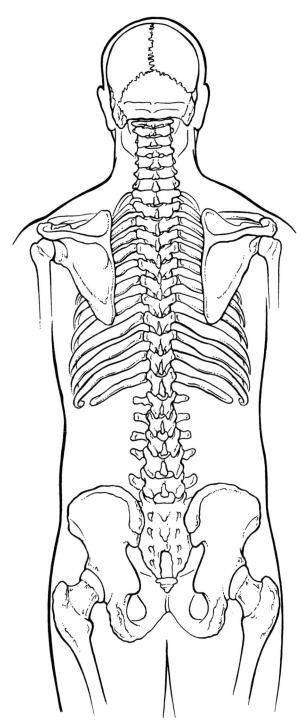

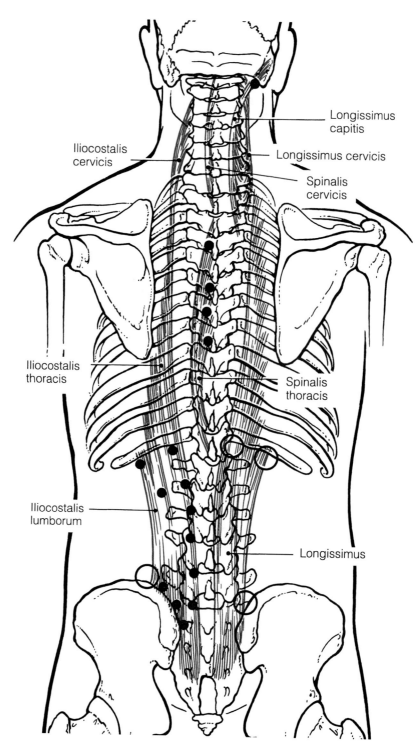

Longissimus
capitis

Iliocostalis
cervicis

Longissimus cervicis

Spinalis
cervicis

Iliocostalis
thoracis

Spinalis
thoracis

Iliocostalis
lumborum

Longissimus

O Important areas to treat.

the posterior median furrow lies between. Note that they lie deep to the superficial extrinsic muscles (*trapezius, latissimus dorsi, levator scapulae,* and *rhomboids*) and to the intermediate extrinsic muscles (*serratus posterior superior* and *inferior*). The intrinsic muscles are in three layers:

Superficial layer
This consists of the *splenius capitis* and *cervicis.*

Intermediate layer
The **erector spinae** (*sacrospinalis*) is the largest muscular mass of the back. It runs vertically from the pelvis to the skull in three columns—the *iliocostalis,* the *longissimus,* and the *spinalis*:

The **iliocostalis** is a three-part muscle. The *iliocostalis lumborum* originates from the iliac crest and inserts into the inferior 6 ribs; the *iliocostalis thoracis* arises from the inferior 6 ribs to insert into the angles of the superior 6 ribs; the *iliocostalis cervicis* ascends from the 3–6 ribs and inserts into the transverse processes of the C6–C4 vertebrae.

The *longissimus* muscle originates from the iliac crest. It is also in three parts. The *longissimus thoracis* inserts into the tips of the transverse processes of all the thoracic vertebrae and into the lower 10 ribs between their tubercles and angles; the *longissimus cervicis* inserts into the posterior tubercles of the transverse processes of C2–C6; the *longissimus capitis* inserts into the mastoid process of the temporal bone.

The **spinalis muscle** is also in three parts: *spinalis thoracis, spinalis cervicis,* and *spinalis capitis.* It arises from the spinous processes in the dorsolumbar regions and inserts into the spinous processes in the upper thoracic region.

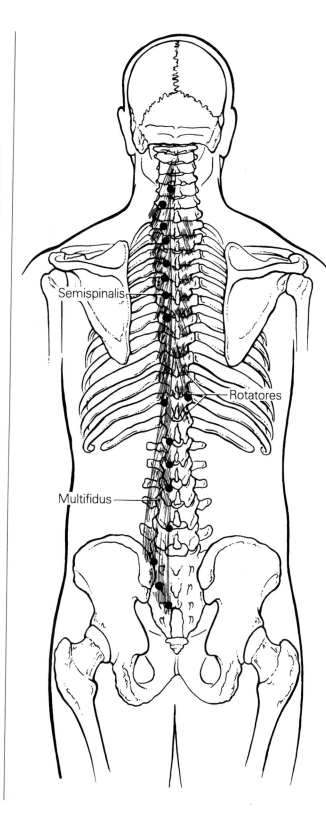

Deep layer

This consists of the transversospinal muscles: the *semispinalis*, the *multifidus*, and the *rotatores*. This group of obliquely-disposed short muscles runs from the transverse processes to the spinous processes of most vertebrae, hence, "transversospinal".

The *semispinalis* muscle, as its name indicates, originates from about half the upper spine (T10 and up) to insert into the thoracic spinous processes (*semispinalis thoracis*), the cervical spinous processes (*semispinalis cervicis*), and the occipital bone (*semispinalis capitis*). The *semispinalis capitis* forms the largest muscle mass in the neck.

The *multifidus* ("many-cleaved") muscle is divided into many bundles that occupy the groove on each side of the spinous processes. These extend the entire length of the spine, but are more substantial in the lower half. The bundles arise from the sacrum and the mammillary processes of L5 to T12, the transverse processes of the thoracic vertebrae, and the articular processes of cervical vertebrae. They ascend over 2–5 vertebrae and insert into the spinous processes.

The *rotatores* are short muscles that arise from the transverse process of one vertebra and insert into the base of the spinous process of the vertebra above.

TREATMENT

Position of patient

Position the patient prone, using a shallow pillow to support the abdomen, thus straightening the lumbar curvature. Allow the arms to hang down freely on the sides of the couch, thus pulling the scapulae laterally.

As a supplementary position, have the patient lie on one side, with hips flexed. This semiprone position allows good access to the quadratus lumborum and lateral aspect of the iliac crest.

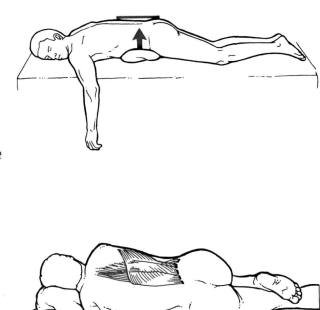

For lumbago, acupuncture is, in acute cases, the most efficient treatment. Needles of from three to four inches in length (ordinary bonnet needles, sterilized, will do) are thrust into the lumbar muscles at the seat of pain, and withdrawn after five or ten minutes. In many instances the relief of pain is immediate, and I can corroborate the statements of Ringer, who taught me this practice, as to its extraordinary and prompt effect in many instances. The constant current is sometimes very beneficial.

William Osler (1909) The Principles and Practice of Medicine, 7th edition, D. Appleton and Company, New York and London, p. 397.

Choice of needle

The minimum length is 2 inches. In the low back and buttock, a 3-inch needle is generally required to penetrate thicker muscles. Since many muscles require treatment, the use of a plunger-type needle holder is often more convenient than individual needles. If individual needles are preferred, a number of them (e.g. eight) may be inserted into selected muscles and left for several minutes (sometimes up to 20 minutes) until muscle shortening is released. The needles are then withdrawn and, if desired, reinserted into other muscles.

Procedure

Treatment of the lumbar back usually includes the intrinsic muscles of the back, the buttocks, and part of the posterior abdominal wall (*quadratus*

BACK • LUMBAR BACK

lumborum and *obliquus externus* and *internus* muscles) on both sides. **Even when there is no pain in the lower limbs, muscles in the lower limbs must be treated if they are tender.** These tender muscles belong to the same segmental levels that are involved in the back.

Although pain is commonly localized to the lower segments, the *erector spinae* muscles extend into the skull; **treatment for low back pain should at least extend into the dorsal back.**

Treat one side (generally, the less painful) before the other. Treatment on one side can sometimes, by reflex stimulation, partially desensitize the other side. Also, any objective changes as they occur in the treated side (e.g. return of lordosis, release of muscle spasm, lessening of tenderness, and improved skin temperature) can be compared to the untreated side.

Needle the attachments of the *obliquus externus* and *internus*, *latissimus dorsi*, *quadratus lumborum*, *iliocostalis lumborum*, and *longissimus thoracis* at about ½ inch superior to the iliac crest.

Palpate and needle the *erector spinae* muscular column at each segmental level from L1 to L5, the *spinalis* about ½ inch from the midline, the *longissimus thoracis* about 1 inch from the midline, and the *iliocostalis lumborum* about 2 inches from the midline. Insert the needle perpendicularly when close to the midline (A) and **angle it medially as insertion moves away from the midline** (B).

Palpate the muscles above L1 in the dorsal back, as they may be tender and also require needling. When needling has produced relaxation in the muscles of the

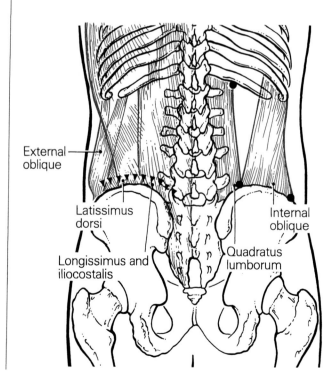

External oblique

Latissimus dorsi

Longissimus and iliocostalis

Internal oblique

Quadratus lumborum

superficial and intermediate layers, the needle is reinserted through the *longissimus* muscle to reach muscles of the deep layer (the *semispinalis* and *rotatores*) but, if there is no spasm in the first layer, both layers may be needled simultaneously.

The "super-contracture"

When paraspinal muscles at consecutive segmental levels are needled, resistance to needle penetration may be substantially increased at the involved level(s) when compared to the segments above and below.

Occasionally, the needle encounters a contracture that seems bony-hard and cannot be penetrated to the depth reached at other levels. Penetration, then, may only be possible by applying some considerable force, and after repeated "pecking".

Finally, when the needle enters the dense, fibrotic contracture, the patient experiences the intense cramp described previously. This gradually diminishes as the needle-grasp is liberated. **The dense, fibrotic contracture is an important and crucial clinical finding which is invisible to radiological, CAT, or MRI techniques and may be labelled as the "invisible lesion".**

However, the hard contracture is but a consequence of Cannon's law. Cannon described four types of increased sensitivity:

1. Superduration of response, where the amplitude of responses is unchanged, but their course is prolonged.
2. Hyperexcitability, where the threshold for the stimulating agent is lower than normal.
3. Increased susceptibility, where lessened stimuli that do not have

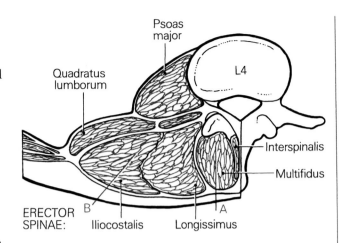

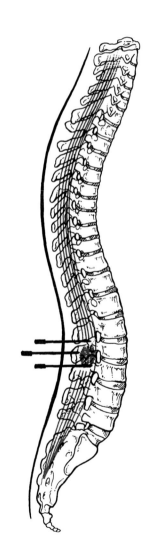

to exceed a threshold produce responses of normal amplitude.

4. Super-reactivity, where the ability of the tissue to respond is augmented. The hard contracture may thus represent a "super-contracture", of superduration, in a super-reactive and super-excitable muscle.

Re-palpate the above muscles after needling. Compare the treated side (which should be relaxed and less tender) with the other.

Lower limb

Buttock

EXAMINATION

Identify landmarks

Locate the greater tuberosity of the femur; the iliac crest (its highest point, as palpated posteriorly, is at the level of the fourth lumbar vertebra); the anterior superior iliac spine; the tubercle of the crest (located about 5 cm posteriorly); the posterior superior iliac spine, which may be difficult to palpate, but skin and underlying fascia are attached to it and form skin dimples. A line joining these dimples crosses the second sacral vertebra at the middle of the sacroiliac joints.

Surface markings

The superior gluteal nerve: the junction of the upper and middle third of a line between the posterior superior iliac spine and the top of the greater trochanter is the point where the superior gluteal nerve and vessels leave the pelvis. The *piriformis* muscle is immediately inferior to these. The sciatic nerve passes from under the cover of the *gluteus maximus* about midway between the ischial tuberosity and the greater trochanter. The sciatic nerve leaves the pelvis with the internal pudendal vessels and the pudendal nerve below the point of emergence of the superior gluteal nerve, separated by the width of the *piriformis* muscle.

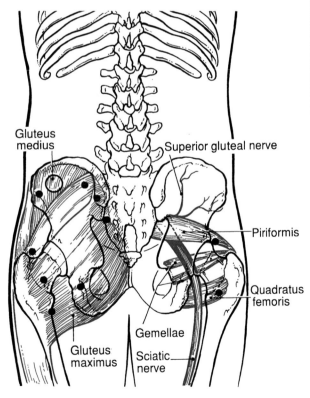

Gluteus medius

Superior gluteal nerve

Piriformis

Quadratus femoris

Gemellae

Gluteus maximus

Sciatic nerve

O The gluteus medius is tender in most back and leg conditions and requires treatment.

TREATMENT

Treatment of the buttock always includes treatment to both sides of the back.

Position of patient

Place the patient in the supplementary position, lying on one side with the upper hip flexed. (The ischial tuberosity is covered by the *gluteus maximus* when the hip is extended, but is palpable when the hip is flexed.)

Palpate and needle the tender bands in the gluteus maximus muscle (the small area on the outer surface of the ilium between the posterior gluteal line and iliac crest, back of the sacrum and sacrotuberous ligament to the iliotibial tract of the fascia lata and gluteal tuberosity above the *linea aspera*).

Needle the gluteus medius muscle (the outer surface of the ilium between the iliac crest and middle gluteal line to the lateral surface of the greater trochanter along a line downward and forward at about 2 inches from the iliac crest).

Then, needle these muscles as they insert into the greater trochanter and iliotibial tract.

When the gluteal muscles are relaxed, the *quadratus femoris, gluteus medius*, and *gemelli* muscles can be palpated. Needle these muscles at about 2 inches from the greater trochanter.

The *gluteus minimus* muscle (the outer surface of the ilium between middle and inferior gluteal lines to the impression on anterior part of the greater trochanter) can be needled through the *medius*.

The sciatic nerve runs deep to the gluteus maximus muscle, midway between the greater trochanter and ischial tuberosity. In IMS, when no medications are injected, no serious harm will result from accidentally piercing the sciatic nerve. But to avoid the sciatic nerve, needle close to the greater trochanter and ischial tuberosity.

"Ischial bursitis" ("Tailor's bottom")

A not unusual complaint is pain in the region of the ischial tuberosity on sitting. To treat, flex the hip and needle the gluteus maximus and the muscles which arise from the ischial tuberosity close to their origins—the adductor magnus, semitendinosus, semimembranosus, and biceps (long head) (see Posterior thigh, p. 90).

For pain in the buttocks, it is important to treat the deep space between the medial aspect of the iliac crest and the sacrum where the multifidus originates.

Fascia lata fasciitis

When there is shortening in the gluteus maximus muscle, there is generally also shortening in the tensor fasciae latae muscle (from the anterior superior iliac spine to the iliotibial tract), and tightening in the fascia lata. A dull ache develops in the low back that extends through the lateral hip into the thigh. There can be pain over the trochanter, i.e. "trochanteric bursitis".

Iliotibial band friction syndrome

The fascia lata ends at the iliotibial tract at the lateral condyle of the tibia, and friction can be caused by shortening of the gluteus maximus and tensor fasciae latae muscles. Treat by needling tender points in these muscles, as well as in the vastus lateralis.

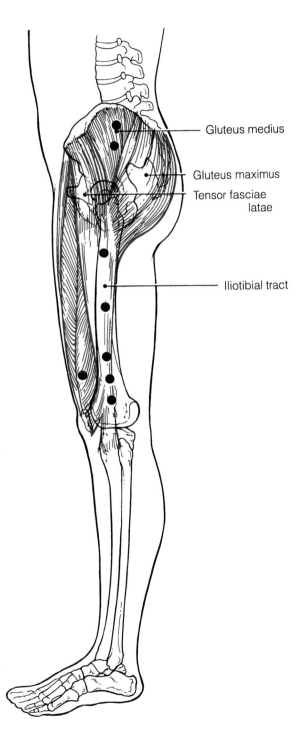

Gluteus medius

Gluteus maximus

Tensor fasciae latae

Iliotibial tract

LOWER LIMB • BUTTOCK

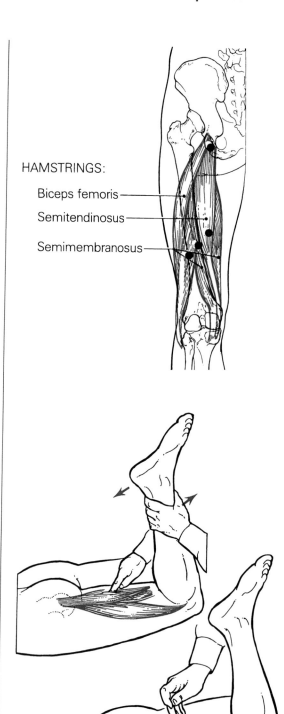

HAMSTRINGS:

Biceps femoris

Semitendinosus

Semimembranosus

Posterior thigh

EXAMINATION

Three large muscles make up the hamstrings: the *semimembranosus, semitendinosus,* and *biceps femoris.* They have a common origin from the ischial tuberosity deep to the *gluteus maximus,* and run to the proximal ends of tibia and fibula.

Biceps femoris: long head from the medial part of the ischial tuberosity with the semitendinosus; short head from the linea aspera to the head of the fibula.

Semitendinosus: from the medial part of the ischial tuberosity to the medial surface of the tibia below the knee joint.

Semimembranosus: from the lateral part of the ischial tuberosity to the posterior surface of the medial condyle of the tibia deep to the medial ligament of the knee joint.

These muscles extend the hip and flex the knee, and are therefore examined and treated when there is pain in either of these joints.

TREATMENT

Treatment of the hamstrings always includes the intrinsic muscles of the back. Likewise, lumbar spondylosis may manifest as pain in the hamstrings. In low back pain, tender hamstrings are always treated. To demonstrate the muscles, the knee is flexed at 90 degrees against resistance. Needle the tender midportion of each muscle; but further needle insertions along the length of the muscles may be necessary to produce full relaxation.

Anterior thigh and knee

EXAMINATION

Identify bony landmarks

Locate the anterior superior iliac spine and the pubic tubercle.

Surface markings

The femoral artery begins at a point midway between the anterior superior iliac spine and the pubic symphysis. Draw a line from that point to the adductor tubercle; the proximal two thirds of that line represents the femoral artery. The continuation is the popliteal artery: a line down the center of the popliteal fossa to the level of the tubercle of the tibia. Anterior tibial artery: a point midway between the tubercle of the tibia and the head of the fibula to midway between the two malleoli. Dorsalis pedis artery: a line continued to the proximal part of the first intermetatarsal space.

Avoid the femoral triangle which contains the femoral vessels and the femoral nerve, bounded laterally by the sartorius, and medially by the medial margin of the adductor longus; its floor is formed by the *iliopsoas*, *pectineus*, and *adductor longus*.

Muscles

Pectineus: from the pectineal line of the pubis and the surface in front of it to a line from the lesser trochanter to the linea aspera.

Gracilis: from the outer surface of the inferior pubic ramus to the medial side of the upper end of the tibia.

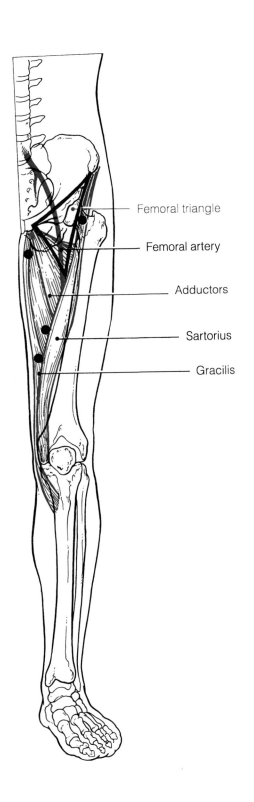

Femoral triangle

Femoral artery

Adductors

Sartorius

Gracilis

Adductor longus: from the anterior surface of the body of pubis in the angle between the crest and the symphysis to the linea aspera.

Adductor brevis: from the outer surface of the inferior pubic ramus to the linea aspera.

Adductor magnus: from the inferior pubic ramus and lower part of the ischial tuberosity to the gluteal tuberosity, linea aspera, medial supra-condylar line, and adductor tubercle.

These are important muscles to treat because L2 is a frequently injured segmental level. Always check the Fabere sign. Very often these muscles are shortened when the patient is under stress. Sometimes a cervical spine disorder cannot be treated without releasing the adductors. They are also responsible for pain in the hip—as often as not, pain in the buttock and hip can be caused by shortening in the adductors. They are also responsible for pain in the hip in osteoarthritis.

TREATMENT

Pain in the groin

This is often associated with shortening of the above muscles. The Fabere sign may be positive, i.e. there is pain on attempted flexion, abduction, external rotation, and extension. Treat the above muscles, but dorsolumbar paraspinal muscles, especially the erector spinae muscles at L2–3, also must be treated.

Pain in the pubis

Shortening of the adductor muscles commonly causes pain at the anterior aspect of the pubis. Treat the above muscles. With the patient supine, place the leg to be treated in the

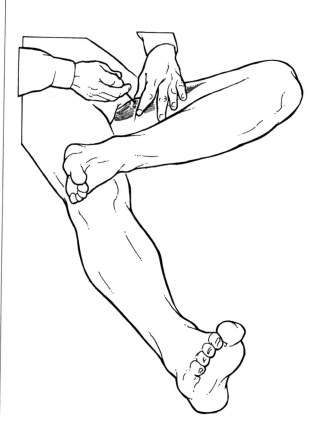

Fabere position, stretching the adductor muscles. Needle the muscles about two inches from their origin (gripping the muscles between thumb and index finger) and again at about 2–3 inches from their insertion.

HLA-B27 spinal arthropathies

If the Fabere test is forced and there is pain in the sacroiliac joint, "sacroiliitis" is suspected. Sacroiliitis presents in young people (usually men in the same family) who may be HLA-B27 positive. Disorders belonging to this category of spinal arthropathies include ankylosing spondylitis, Reiter's disease, and reactive, psoriatic, colitic, and juvenile arthritis. The arthritis may be associated with aortitis, iritis, or a recent history of sexually transmitted infection (gonorrhea or Chlamydia). Although IMS cannot change the condition, the shortened muscles in these patients can respond to maintenance treatment.

Examination of the sacroiliac joint

Contrary to popular belief, this joint allows slight movement. To check: with the patient erect, the examiner places one finger on the posterior superior iliac spine on one side; another finger is placed on the sacrum, opposite to and level with the first finger. The patient is asked to stand on the leg on that side, and fully flex the other hip. Normally, there is a slight movement in the sacroiliac joint, and the finger tips move apart by about ½ inch.

The "piriformis syndrome"

The *piriformis* muscle (the pelvic surface of the sacrum from the 2nd to

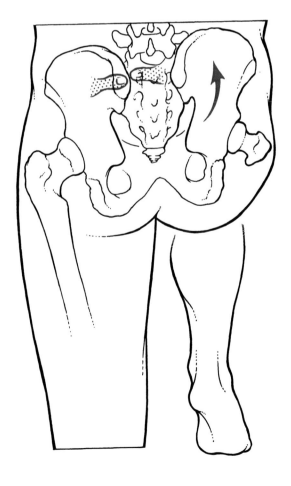

4th segments lateral to the anterior sacral foramina to the top of the greater trochanter, the muscle passing out of the pelvis through the greater sciatic foramen) fills the greater sciatic foramen. When shortened, the muscle can sometimes compress the sciatic nerve and cause pain in its distribution.

The "piriformis syndrome" is suspected when there is point tenderness in the sciatic notch, as well as during rectal examination. To test, place hands on the lateral aspect of the seated patient's knees. There is pain and weakness on abduction against resistance.

Rarely, the muscle can also become tender, and is the site of pain in sacro-iliitis. The muscle can be palpated and needled through the *gluteus maximus* after the latter is relaxed.

Knee pain

Knee pain is commonly caused by shortening in muscles that activate the joint. These muscles are innervated by segmental nerves from the lumbar spine; therefore, examination and treatment of the knee always includes the back, where L2–3, 3–4 and 4–5 are usually found to be involved.

Knee flexors
Two on the lateral side:

Biceps femoris (long head from the medial part of the ischial tuberosity, short head from the linea aspera to the head of the fibula).

Popliteus (lateral condyle of the femur to the tibia above the soleal line).

Four on the medial side (pes anserinus):

Sartorius (the anterior superior iliac spine and outer edge of the iliac crest for 2 inches to the medial side of the upper end of the tibia).

Gracilis (the outer surface of the inferior pubic ramus to the medial side of upper end of tibia).

Semitendinosus.

Semimembranosus.

With knee flexed and leg at a right angle to thigh, sartorius insertion is placed anteriorly, gracilis intermediate, and semitendinosus posteriorly.

Medial knee joint pain

Shortening of the above muscles is a common cause of pain in the medial aspect of the knee; the knee usually cannot fully extend. Releasing the shortened muscles relieves medial joint pain, and improves range, sometimes within minutes, even when there is a minor tear of the medial meniscus (without locking). With knee flexed, the muscles are needled at their musculotendinous junctions, about two inches above the medial joint line.

Knee extensors

Pain in the anterior aspect of the knee is commonly caused by shortening of the knee extensors. The quadriceps femoris consists of four muscles:

Rectus femoris has two heads (the anterior inferior iliac spine, the groove above the acetabulum).

Vastus lateralis (the base of the greater trochanter, the line to the linea aspera, the lateral lip of the linea aspera).

Vastus medialis (the lower half of the anterior intertrochanteric line, the spiral line, the medial lip of the linea aspera).

Vastus intermedius (the proximal ⅔ of the anterior and lateral surfaces of the shaft of the femur).

These four muscles join the

Treating the **pes anserinus**, the tendinous expansion and attachment of the *sartorius*, *gracilis*, and *semitendinosus*.

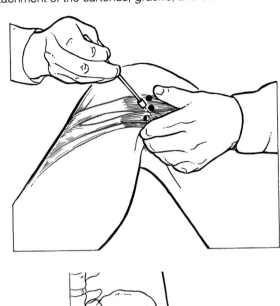

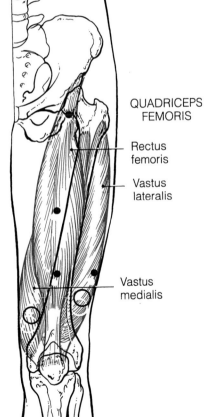

QUADRICEPS FEMORIS

Rectus femoris

Vastus lateralis

Vastus medialis

O Important areas to treat for medial joint line pain and lateral knee pain.

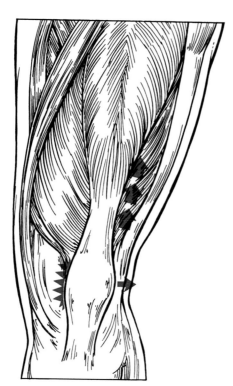

common extensor tendon which is inserted into the patella. From the lower margin of the patella, the insertion is continued by the ligamentum patellae to the tubercle of the tibia.

Patellofemoral pain

Shortening of the knee extensors increases patellofemoral loading, and can cause knee pain, e.g. the patellofemoral pain syndrome. The patient is often aware of crepitus (a creaking feeling behind the patella, especially when squatting) and a feeling of stiffness.

Chondromalacia patellae

Shortening also causes misalignment and pathologic lesions in the articular surface of the patella. These usually begin in the medial facet. Softening and swelling of the cartilage is followed by fragmentation and fissuring and, eventually, erosion of the cartilage to the bone.

This common, but much misunderstood condition responds to needling of the quadriceps femoris, but the upper lumbar paraspinal muscles are always involved and must be treated to free the nerve roots.

Leg and dorsum of foot

EXAMINATION

The paraspinal muscles of the low back must also be examined and treated when there is pain in the muscles of the leg. Likewise, when there is low back pain, the leg muscles are examined.

Muscles on anterior aspect

Tibialis anterior: proximal ⅔ of the tibia to the medial cuneiform and base of 1st metatarsal. This long, thick muscle lies along the lateral surface of the tibia and is easy to palpate. A foot drop may occur from injury to the common peroneal nerve (or its branch, the deep peroneal nerve), or from compression of the L5 nerve root. A partial foot drop from L5 radiculopathy may respond to needling of the muscle.

Extensor digitorum longus: the proximal ⅔ of the fibula to the extensor expansions of four lateral toes.

Extensor hallucis longus: the fibula deep to the extensor digitorum longus to the base of the distal phalanx of the big toe.

Extensor digitorum brevis: the upper surface of the calcaneum to four tendons; the medial tendon, the extensor hallucis brevis, goes to the base of the proximal phalanx of the big toe, crossing over the dorsalis pedis artery; the other three tendons join the extensor expansions of the 2nd, 3rd and 4th toes.

Peroneus tertius: the distal ⅓ of the fibula to the base of the 5th metatarsal.

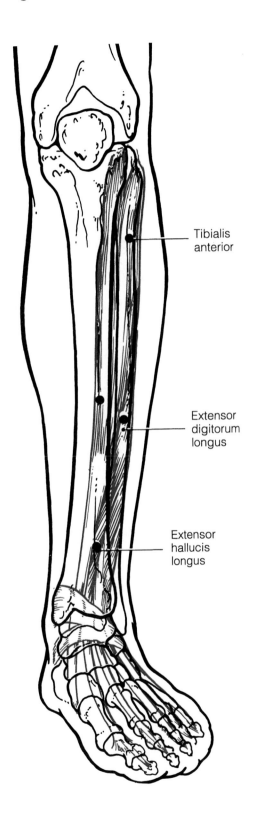

Tibialis anterior

Extensor digitorum longus

Extensor hallucis longus

LOWER LIMB • LEG AND DORSUM OF FOOT

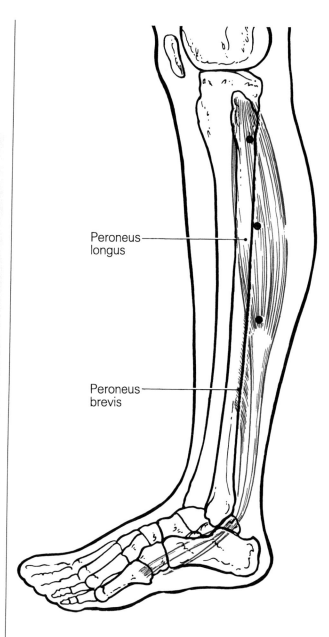

Peroneus longus

Peroneus brevis

Muscles on lateral side

Peroneus longus: the proximal two thirds of the fibula to the medial cuneiform and base of the 1st metatarsal.

Peroneus brevis: the distal two thirds of the fibula to the base of the 5th metatarsal. The two tendons lie in a groove at the back of the lateral malleolus.

TREATMENT

"Shin splints"

This is a lay term for a painful condition of the anterior compartment of the leg which occurs following vigorous or lengthy exercise. This overuse condition can occur when ankle dorsiflexors, the tibialis anterior (and extensor hallucis longus and brevis), and sometimes the ankle evertors (peroneus longus and brevis), shorten in the anterior crural compartment and reduce blood flow to the muscles, i.e. "anterior shin splints". Chronic overuse may lead to microtraumata and scar tissue formation. When plantar flexors— the tibialis posterior, flexor hallucis longus, and flexor digitorum longus (see Calf, p. 99)—are painful, the condition is sometimes known as "posterior shin splints".

Tibial stress syndrome

Chronic traction at the attachments of the muscles to bone may result in localized periostitis. (X-rays may be indicated when changes may be positive at the attachments, and a stress fracture may need to be excluded.)

All the above conditions respond to needling of the involved muscles.

Compare range of plantar flexion and inversion of ankles. In anterior shin splints, forced plantar flexion causes pain in the anterior crural compartment.

Calf

EXAMINATION

Treatment of calf pain always includes an examination of the low back, as pain in the calf is a common manifestation of lumbar spondylosis.

Superficial muscles of back of leg

Gastrocnemius: medial and lateral heads from the posterior aspect of the femur just above the condyles.

Soleus is deep to the gastrocnemius: from the proximal ⅓ of the fibula, soleal line of tibia, and fibrous arch across the popliteal vessels near their bifurcation.

The muscles unite to form the tendo calcaneus, which is inserted into the calcaneum. **Shortening of these muscles strains the tendo calcaneus and causes Achilles tendonitis.**

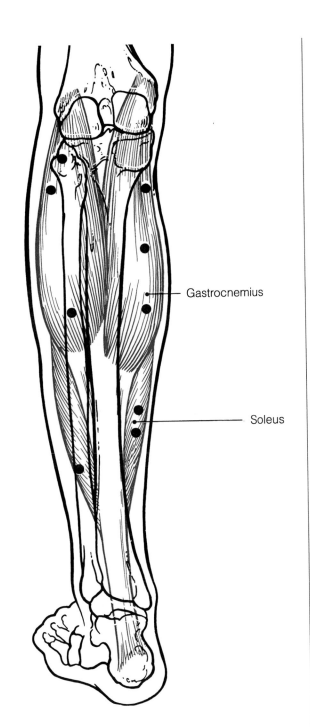

Gastrocnemius

Soleus

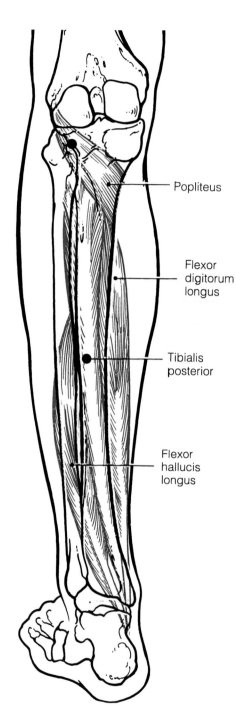

Popliteus

Flexor
digitorum
longus

Tibialis
posterior

Flexor
hallucis
longus

Deep muscles of back of leg

Popliteus: the lateral condyle of the femur to the tibia above the soleal line.

Flexor hallucis longus: the fibula to the base of the distal phalanx of the big toe.

Flexor digitorum longus: the tibia to the four tendons in the foot.

Tibialis posterior: the tibia and fibula to the tuberosity of the navicular with slips to all the bones of the tarsus, except the talus, and to the base of the middle metatarsal bones.

TREATMENT

Pain in the back of the knee may result from shortening in the popliteus muscle.

Pain in the lateral side of the leg above the lateral malleolus. Calf pain nearly always includes pain and tenderness in the peroneus longus and brevis.

Pain in the medial side of the leg above the medial malleolus. Calf pain is often associated with pain and tenderness in the flexor digitorum longus.

Tenosynovitis

Shortening of the tendons of the *tibialis anterior, tibialis posterior, extensor digitorum longus,* or *peroneal* muscles may cause pain similar to De Quervain's tenosynovitis at the wrist. Release of the involved shortened muscles relieves the condition.

Achilles tendonitis

Release the soleus and gastrocnemii muscles. When pain is bilateral, treat one side at a time only as soreness from needling can cause limping.

Treatment of any condition in the lower limb requires muscles on both anterior and posterior aspects to be freed. Check range of joints before and after treatment.

Foot

TREATMENT

Arches of the foot

The integrity of the arches of the foot, particularly the medial arch, is maintained by the action of the *tibialis posterior*, *flexor hallucis longus*, and *flexor digitorum longus* muscles through the bracing action of their tendons. These muscles must be examined and treated in the calf when there is pain in the foot.

Pain on the medial aspect of the foot

This can be from shortening of the *tibialis anterior* muscle pulling on its attachment at the medial surface of the medial cuneiform and base of the first metatarsal bones. Treatment is to the muscle in the leg.

Hallux valgus

Shortening of the *extensor hallucis longus* and *extensor hallucis brevis* muscles can cause lateral deviation of the big toe, and produce medial deviation of the head of the first metatarsal. A bunion can form at the medial aspect of the metatarso-phalangeal joint. In the early stage, before severe arthritic damage to the joint occurs, the condition responds to needling of these muscles, and alignment of the toe can return to normal after a few treatments.

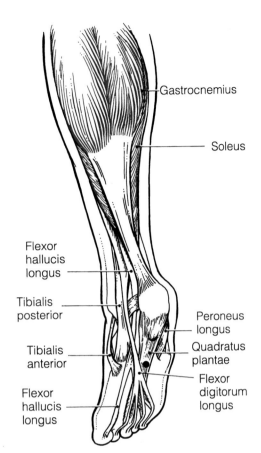

Gastrocnemius

Soleus

Flexor hallucis longus

Tibialis posterior

Tibialis anterior

Flexor hallucis longus

Peroneus longus

Quadratus plantae

Flexor digitorum longus

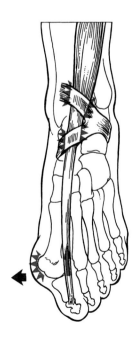

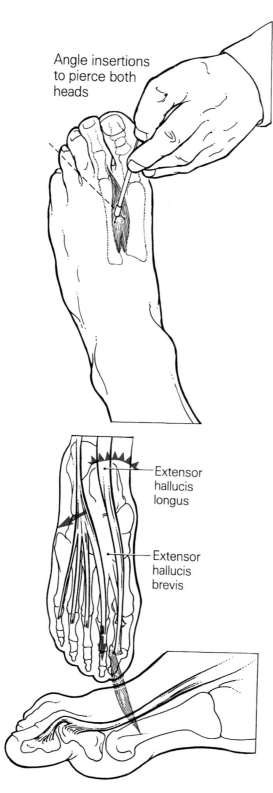

Angle insertions to pierce both heads

Extensor hallucis longus

Extensor hallucis brevis

Hallux rigidus

Degenerative joint disease may occur in the first metatarso-phalangeal joint, causing pain, tenderness, and stiffness (often bilateral). Early cases respond to needling of the first dorsal *interossei* muscle. The Matchstick test usually yields deep indentations. Using a 1-inch long needle, pierce the muscle between the first and second metatarsals at the most tender areas (about 1½ inches proximal to the heads of the metatarsals). The *flexor hallucis longus* and *brevis* and *extensor hallucis longus* muscles may also require treatment.

Pain in the sole

This may result from:

Shortening of the *extensor hallucis longus* and *extensor digitorum longus* muscles which dorsiflex the toes, thus angulating the metatarso-phalangeal joint and exposing the tender under-side of the heads of metatarsals and plantar nerves to pressure on walking.

Metatarsalgia. Pain in the metatarsal region may arise from weakness of the intrinsic muscles. Palpate for tenderness in the flexor digiti minimi, abductor digiti minimi, flexor digitorum brevis, flexor hallucis brevis, abductor hallucis, and adductor hallucis muscles. Also check the flexor hallucis longus and flexor digitorum longus muscles in the calf.

Plantar (Morton's) neuralgia. An interdigital plantar neuroma may subsequently develop in the inter-digital nerves, commonly between the third and fourth toes, causing pain, numbness, tingling, aching, and burning in the distal forefoot. Treatment is to the above extensor muscles. The long flexors and lumbricals may also require treatment if tender (see below).

Plantar fasciitis is one of the most common causes of foot pain. The condition is frequently associated with systemic rheumatoid diseases, and many patients are HLA-B27 positive and have other tender muscles in the body. A hallmark for diagnosis is point tenderness along the longitudinal bands of the plantar fascia. Identify and needle the discrete points of tenderness, penetrating through to reach the *flexor digitorum brevis* and *flexor accessorius* muscles (*quadratus plantae*).

Calcaneal heel spur which sometimes develops from long-standing plantar fasciitis, responds to the same treatment. Direct needling of the spur is seldom necessary.

Important—when there are symptoms on both sides, treat only one side at a time as the patient may limp for a day or so!

LOWER LIMB • FOOT

Part 3

Supplementary information

Musculoskeletal pain of spondylotic origin

A PROPOSED MODEL AND TREATMENT RATIONALE

C. Chan Gunn MD, A. E. Sola MD, J. D. Loeser MD, C. R. Chapman PhD

INTRODUCTION

Chronic pain problems of obscure origin are frequently seen, poorly understood, difficult to diagnose, and rarely treated successfully by medical intervention. Clearly, new approaches to the diagnosis and treatment of such problems are needed. Medical diagnosis traditionally presumes that pain is a signal of tissue injury—nociception or inflammation—that is conveyed to the CNS via a healthy nervous system. However, when there is abnormal physiology in nerve and muscle, irritative manifestations (including some types of pain and involuntary activity in muscle) can arise.[1,24] Our clinical experience leads us to postulate that there is a large group of patients whose chronic musculoskeletal pain may be the result of abnormal physiology in nerve and muscle consequent to neuropathy, that is, a disturbance of function and/or pathological change in the nerve.[3] These pain syndromes display abnormal sensorimotor phenomena and appear to share a common pathophysiology of impulses generated abnormally by excitable nerve and muscle membranes.[5,10,14,17,26,27,28] Our propositions are supported by clinical observations that these syndromes lack evidence of ongoing nociception or inflammation, but are generally accompanied by subtle motor, sensory, or autonomic signs of neuropathy that disappear as the pain resolves.

Our neuropathy model for chronic pain attempts to explain this group of so-called idiopathic pain syndromes as other models such as the gate theory can not. Whereas the gate model would account for degenerative chronic pain in terms of the different proportions of large to small fibers remaining after nerve degeneration, the neuropathy concept would suggest abnormal activity arising from irritation or damage to a peripheral nerve, and related secondary effects on associated muscles, joints, and other tissues.

PHASES OF PAIN: IMMEDIATE, ACUTE, AND CHRONIC

Wall has described pain as a general reaction pattern of three sequential and natural behavioral phases: immediate (nociception), acute (inflammatory), and chronic.[25] Since each phase may exist independently or in any combination and proportion with the others, for present purposes they are regarded as distinct physiologic entities rather than facets of a single entity. *Chronic pain* may result from ongoing nociception/inflammation, psychologic factors, or functional and structural alterations within the central or peripheral nervous systems. Our discussion represents the last category and centers on a large group of musculoskeletal pain syndromes for which we postulate a physiological basis (Table I, p. 115).

MUSCULOSKELETAL PAIN AS A RESULT OF NEUROPATHY

We postulate that there can be several possible mechanisms by which neuropathy can cause musculoskeletal pain, including:

- In neuropathy, *the normal efferent flow of impulses to nerves and muscles is diminished,* which can cause excitable nerve and muscle membranes to *generate anomalous impulses.* These impulses may proceed along nociceptive pathways to evoke abnormal sensorimotor activity including pain and muscle shortening.
- *Muscle shortening* can cause pain by *compressing intramuscular nociceptors* that have become supersensitive because of neuropathy.
- *Muscle shortening* in paraspinal muscle can *compress nerve roots* and further irritate them: a vicious circle may be created and neuropathic (i.e. radiculopathic) pain perpetuated.
- *Neuropathy degrades collagen.* Muscle shortening in activity-stressed parts of the body with neuropathy-induced degraded collagen[12] can lead to degenerative changes and pain in tendons and joints.

Abnormal impulse generation

Chronic pain can result when impulses arise abnormally from supersensitive excitable membranes of muscle; that is, their capacity to respond to chemical or mechanical stimuli is exaggerated: the threshold of a stimulus can be lower than normal, the response may be prolonged, and the capacity to respond may be augmented.[2,4,23] Sensitization has been shown to occur in many structures of the body including peripheral nerve, dorsal root ganglion, skeletal and smooth muscle, and spinal neurons. Sensitization may occur at some distance from the original injury and affect target structures and nerve endings.[4]

The normal physiologic properties of nerve and muscle excitable membranes depend upon intact innervation to provide a regulatory or "trophic" effect.[2,4,18,23] Formerly, it was supposed that the development of supersensitivity was due to the loss of a putative trophic factor associated with total denervation or decentralization, i.e. "denervation supersensitivity".[4] Recent evidence, however, supports the idea that any measure which blocks the flow of motor impulses and deprives the effector organ of excitatory input for a period of time, can cause "disuse supersensitivity" in that organ, as well as in associated spinal reflexes.[20]

Trains of impulses along axons and muscle fibers are normal, but repetitive firing is abnormal when ectopic or extemporaneous. Abnormal neurogenic and myogenic impulses arise when changes in the immediate environment around a nerve or muscle provide an electrical or chemical stimulus for impulse generation. Anomalous or ectopic impulses then proceed along normal nociceptive pathways to evoke abnormal sensorimotor activity.

Discussion of the many possible mechanisms for abnormal impulse generation (e.g. development of extra-junctional acetylcholine receptors, changes in ion channels, membrane capacitance, voltage-dependent channel gating, current-dependent mechanisms, axon sprouts, ephaptic transmission, and others) is outside the scope of this paper. These were the focus of a recent meeting of scientists and clinicians in which numerous syndromes caused by abnormal discharges were identified.[5] One condition, classified as "sciaticas and brachialgias", corresponds to the type of pain discussed in this paper —"recurrent pain referred to the territory of spinal nerve roots, characterized by clear mechano-sensitivity, usually resulting from focal damage caused by a space-occupying lesion" at "dorsal root fibers (or ganglion cells?)".

For pain to become a symptom, the affected fibers must have pre-existing minor chronic damage or neuropathy; an acute injury to a healthy dorsal root does not produce a sustained discharge.[6] Pain may then be triggered by a new episode of neural damage. In contrast, acute structural deformation of a healthy nerve is not painful or only briefly so. Probably the most common cause of neuropathy is spondylosis (i.e. radiculopathy). Since spondylosis increases with age, we view this group of chronic musculoskeletal pain as a manifestation (though not inevitable) of radiculopathy which, itself, is the consequence of age and injury-related degeneration.[22]

Muscle shortening

Muscle shortening from increased muscle tone (possibly associated with abnormal spinal reflexes or super-sensitive peripheral mechanisms) nearly always accompanies neuro-pathic musculoskeletal pain syndromes. Shortening can cause pain by compressing intramuscular nociceptors that may have become overly sensitive and prone to abnormal impulse generation.

Long-standing muscle tension eventually leads to fibrosis and contracture formation. These are usually pain-free, but may become tender and painful if their nociceptors are supersensitive.[16] Travell and Simons have hypothesized that focal areas of tenderness and pain in shortened muscles (trigger points) begin with transient muscle overload that disrupts the sarcoplasmic reticulum and causes it to release calcium ions. These react with ATP and activate the actinomyosin contractile mechanism. Contractures are then maintained by a vicious circle which includes the accumulation of metabolites, vasoconstriction, depletion of ATP, and disruption of the calcium pump.[21] Although transient muscle overload may disrupt sarcoplasmic reticulum, according to our neuropathy model it is probable that the integrity of skeletal muscle has already suffered from the effects of neuropathy,[12] thus predisposing the muscle to overload.

Sustained shortening in paraspinal muscles acting across an inter-vertebral disc space can compress the disc, narrow the intervertebral foramina, and perpetuate the irritation of nerve roots. This self-perpetuating predicament is central to our model.

Secondary pain from tissue degradation

Muscle shortening mechanically stresses ligaments, tendons, cartilage, and bone. When stress occurs in structures that have collagen already weakened as a consequence of neuropathy, the overload can produce degeneration and secondary pain, for example, tendonitis, epicondylitis, spondylosis, discogenic disease, and osteoarthritis among others. When joint integrity is destroyed, pain may be a combination of ongoing nociception (e.g. bone wearing upon bone without intervening cartilage) and neuropathic pain.

CLINICAL PRESENTATION

The clinical manifestations of neuropathy—mixed sensorimotor and autonomic disturbances—have been discussed in the Introduction. Despite the many causes of peripheral neuropathy, their repertoire of clinical manifestations is relatively limited. This is because their pathology is similar: axonal degeneration and/or segmental demyelination with variable degrees of damage and reversibility, from neurapraxia to axonotmesis and neurotmesis.[3] The cardinal feature that differentiates neuropathic pain from inflammatory pain is that affected parts are perceptibly colder.

IMPLICATION FOR DIAGNOSIS AND TREATMENT

Since the mechanisms of neuropathic pain are different from nociception or inflammation, diagnosis and treatment require different approaches. The history usually gives little assistance: often pain arises spontaneously, or the degree of reported pain far exceeds that of the injury. Laboratory, radiological, and routine electrodiagnostic tests are generally unhelpful. Diagnosis, therefore, depends on the examiner's acumen and experience. Treatment is also different and depends on the degree and reversibility of neuropathy which can vary considerably. The variety of treatment methods is extensive. Treatment goals are:

- *restoration of diminished efferent impulse flow* allowing supersensitivity and other abnormal features of neuropathy to return to normal,
- *removal of the cause of nerve irritation*, and
- *promotion of healing.*

We propose a hypothesis for the therapeutic mechanism of physical therapies, and that dry needling can provide these specified goals:

Restoration of diminished impulse flow

In most injuries, the degree of neuropathy is usually minimal, and pain resolves spontaneously. In other injuries the degree of neuropathy may be minor, and interference to impulse flow is temporary. In these cases, a short-term replacement for diminished impulse flow may be all that is necessary to relieve pain, pending recovery of the nerve. This may be achieved by substituting another form of excitatory input to stimulate or "exercise" the deprived organ.[20] For example, development of supersensitivity in denervated glands has been prevented by "exercising" the gland with daily injection of pilocarpine; also, features of denervation in skeletal muscle have been reversed by direct electrical stimulation of the deprived muscle.[15]

In a similar way, the local application of various forms of physical modalities may temporarily maintain the physiologic integrity of deprived structures by augmenting the reduced trophic factor. In physical therapies, the different stimulus modalities are sensed by their specific receptors, transduced into nerve impulses, and relayed to the spinal cord. As with the patellar reflex, stimulation reaches the affected part indirectly. It is the reflex response in efferent fibers to the affected structure that stimulates the therapeutic target.

Thus, physical therapies can provide relief while the nerve heals (usually within days or, at the most, weeks). Unfortunately, external forms of reflex stimulation are short-lived and cannot furnish long-lasting benefit: when therapy is discontinued, its stimulus ceases. Therefore, when pain persists, treatment with a more effective physical modality is indicated.

We have found that muscle shortening is an inherent component of persistent musculoskeletal pain, and its release is central to treatment. Where simpler measures fail to release muscle shortening, an injection technique generally succeeds. Local anesthetics are commonly employed, but normal physiological saline has also been used with good results.[22] The benefit of injection methods is partly derived from the local inflammation created by the needle regardless of the substance injected: thus, dry needle stimulation, without injected substances, is also effective.[13,22]

One of the body's responses to inflammation is the generation of injury potentials. The insertion of a needle into a muscle generates bursts of electrical discharges with amplitudes as high as 2 mV. These are greatly prolonged in neuropathy (> 300 ms), and are further augmented by manipulation of the needle. These discharges can cause a shortened muscle to visibly fasci-culate and relax instantly or within minutes.[9] Injured tissue also yields current, known as the "current of injury".[8] First described by Galvani in 1797, this current was later measured by Dubois-Reymond in 1860 to be approximately a microampere. Recent measurements[11] using a vibrating probe (which can measure steady extracellular currents as small as 0.1 microamperes/cm^2) showed a freshly amputated finger-tip to generate 500 microampere/cm^2.

Stimulation by needling can reach deep muscles (especially lumbar paraspinal muscles) which are otherwise inaccessible, and its effect can persist for days, until the miniature wounds heal.[9] Pain relief and muscle relaxation in one region can spread to the entire segment, suggesting a reflex mechanism involving spinal modulatory systems. Sympathetic hyperactivity also responds to reflex stimulation, and the relaxation of smooth muscle can spread to the entire segment releasing vasospasm[7] and lympho-constriction.

Removal of the cause of nerve irritation

In spondylosis, efferent flow of impulses is most commonly impeded at the spine where shortened para-spinal muscles compress the nerve. To break this vicious circle, these muscles nearly always require needling.

Promotion of healing

When muscle shortening is associated with extensive fibrosis, another therapeutic mechanism—the healing process—may be involved. Treatment of extensively fibrotic contractures necessitates more exten-sive needling. The progressive nature of symptomatic relief, substantiated by the gradual amelioration of objective clinical findings, suggests that a healing process is involved. Needle injury physically dissipates fibrous tissue, causes local bleeding, and may deliver numerous growth factors to the injured area, including the platelet-derived growth factor (PDGF) which attracts cells, induces DNA synthesis, and stimulates collagen and protein formation.[19] PDGF is a principal mitogen responsible for cell proliferation. Body cells are normally exposed only to a filtrate of plasma (interstitial fluid), and would not see the platelet factor except in the presence of injury, hemorrhage, and blood coagulation. This is a unique benefit not provided by other forms of local treatment.

CONCLUSION

The neuropathy pain model has been proposed as an hypothesis to explain certain chronic musculoskeletal pain problems of seemingly obscure origin and for which there is no effective alternative clinical diagnostic procedure or treatment.

The major points of the model offered are:

- For pain of neural origin to become persistent, pre-existing nerve damage is a prerequisite. Spondylotic radiculopathy is probably the most common cause of nerve damage, and pain is a possible, but not inevitable, manifestation of spondylosis.
- Neuropathy can block the normal efferent flow of motor impulses to nerves and muscles. This, in turn, can cause nerve and muscle membranes to generate anomalous impulses that proceed along conventional pathways to evoke abnormal sensorimotor activity, including pain.
- Muscle shortening invariably

accompanies neuropathy and is an inherent part of musculoskeletal pain.
- Muscle shortening can strain tendinous attachments and upset joint alignment. When superimposed upon neuropathy-induced collagen degradation, it can give rise to degenerative changes that can cause secondary pain.
- The diagnosis of neuropathic pain depends on clinical examination for signs of neuropathy. Laboratory tests give little assistance.
- In lesser degrees of neuropathy, simple physical therapies can provide relief while the nerve heals, probably by substituting for absent impulses with reflex stimulation.
- In persistent pain, the release of muscle shortening is necessary. Muscle shortening responds best to dry needling.
- Dry needling stimulation lasts longer than other forms of physical therapies, probably through the generation of a current-of-injury which can continue for days.
- When paraspinal muscle shortening compresses nerve roots, it must be released.
- Needle stimulation may also provide a unique therapeutic benefit: it can promote healing by releasing a growth factor.

Our model can account for many chronic pain syndromes that the gate theory can not; however, like all models, this one needs challenge and further refinement. Although there is literature to support most of its postulates and assumptions, it is neither intended to be a definitive review nor a final statement on the role of peripheral neuropathy in chronic pain.

REFERENCES

1. Asbury A K, Fields H L 1984 Pain due to peripheral nerve damage: an hypothesis. Neurology (Cleveland) 34: 1587–1590
2. Axelsson J, Thesleff S 1959 A study of supersensitivity in denervated mammalian skeletal muscles. Journal of Physiology 147: 178–193
3. Bradley W G 1974 Disorders of peripheral nerves. Blackwell Scientific Publications, Oxford
4. Cannon W B, Rosenblueth A 1949 The supersensitivity of denervated structures, a law of denervation. MacMillan, New York
5. Culp W J, Ochoa J 1982 Abnormal nerves and muscles as impulse generators. Oxford University Press, New York
6. Dyck P J, Lambert E H, O'Brien P C 1976 Pain in peripheral neuropathy related to rate and kind of fiber degeneration. Neurology 26: 466–471
7. Ernest M, Lee M H H 1985 Sympathetic vasomotor changes induced by manual and electrical acupuncture of the Hoku Point visualized by thermography. Pain 21: 25–34
8. Galvani A 1953 Commentary on electricity: translated by Robert Montraville Green. Elizabeth Licht Publishing, Cambridge
9. Gunn C C 1978 Transcutaneous neural stimulation, acupuncture and the current of injury. American Journal of Acupuncture 6; 3: 191–196
10. Howe J F, Loeser J D, Calvin W H 1977 Mechanosensitivity of dorsal root ganglia and chronically injured axons: a physiological basis for the radicular pain of nerve root compression. Pain 3: 24–41
11. Jaffe L F 1985 Extracellular current measurements with a vibrating probe. TINS December: 517–521
12. Klein L, Dawson M H, Heiple K G 1977 Turnover of collagen in the adult rat after denervation. Journal of Bone and Joint Surgery 59A: 1065–1067
13. Lewit K 1979 The needle effect in the relief of myofascial pain. Pain 6: 83–90
14. Loeser J D, Howe J F 1980 Deafferentation and neuronal injury. In: Lockard J S, Ward A A (eds) Epilepsy: a window to brain mechanisms. Raven Press, New York, pp 123–135
15. Lomo T 1976 The role of activity in the control of membrane and contractile properties of skeletal muscle. In: Thesleff S (ed) Motor innervation of muscle. Academic Press, New York, pp 289–315
16. McCain G 1983 Fibromyositis. Clinical Review 38: 197–207
17. Ochoa J L, Torebjork E, Marchettini P, Sivak M 1985 Mechanisms of neuropathic pain: cumulative observations, new experiments, and further speculation. In: Fields H L, Dubner R, Cervero F (eds) Advances in pain research and therapy, vol 9. Raven Press, New York
18. Purves D 1976 Long term regulation in the vertebrate peripheral nervous system. International review of physiology. Neurophysiology II, vol 10. University Park Press, Baltimore, pp 125–162
19. Ross R, Vogel A 1978 The platelet-derived growth factor. Cell 14: 203–210
20. Sharpless S K 1975 Supersensitivity-like phenomena in the central nervous system. Federation Proceedings, vol 34, no 10, September 1990–1997
21. Simons D G, Travell J 1981 Letter to editor re: myofascial trigger points, a possible explanation. Pain 10: 106–109
22. Sola A E 1984 Treatment of myofascial pain syndrome. In: Benedetti C, Chapman C R, Morrica G (eds) Advances in pain research and therapy, vol 7. Raven Press, New York, pp 467–485
23. Thesleff S, Sellin L C 1980 Denervation supersensitivity. TINS August: 122–126
24. Thomas P K 1984 Symptomatology and differential diagnosis of peripheral neuropathy: clinical features and differential diagnosis. In: Dyck P J, Thomas P K, Lambert E H, Bunge R (eds) Peripheral neuropathy, vol II. W B Saunders, Philadelphia, pp 1169–1190
25. Wall P D 1979 On the relation of injury to pain, the John J Bonica Lecture. Pain 6: 253–264
26. Wall P D 1979 Changes in damaged nerve and their sensory consequences. In: Bonica J J, Liebeskind J C, Albe-Fessard D G (eds) Advances in pain research and therapy, vol 3. Raven Press, New York, pp 39–50
27. Wall P D, Devor J 1983 Sensory afferent impulses originate from dorsal root ganglia as well as from the periphery in normal and nerve injured rats. Pain 17: pp 321–339
28. Willison R G 1982 Spontaneous discharges in motor nerve fibers. In: Culp W J, Ochoa J (eds) Abnormal nerves and muscles impulse generators. Oxford University Press, New York

Table I. Shortened muscles in common syndromes   115

Table I. Shortened muscles in common syndromes

In neuropathy, muscles can shorten from spasm and/or contracture. By compressing muscle nociceptors, shortening can generate primary pain in muscle or, by mechanically overloading tendons, soft tissue attachments, and the joints they activate, cause secondary pain and degenerative changes in these structures. Musculoskeletal pain syndromes are, therefore, of great diversity. In radiculopathy, since muscles of both primary rami are involved, symptoms can appear in peripheral as well as in paraspinal muscles of the same segment, all of which should always be examined. When paraspinal muscles shorten, they can press upon nerve roots and perpetuate radiculopathic pain. Some common syndromes are listed below.

Syndrome	Shortened muscles
Achilles tendonitis	gastrocnemii, soleus
Bicipital tendonitis	biceps brachii
Bursitis, pre-patellar	quadriceps femoris
Capsulitis, shoulder; "frozen shoulder"	all muscles acting on the shoulder, including trapezius, levator scapulae, rhomboidei, pectoralis major, supra- & infraspinati, teres major & minor, subscapularis, deltoid
Cervical fibrositis	cervical paraspinal muscles
Chondromalacia patellae	quadriceps femoris
De Quervain's tenosynovitis	abductor pollicis longus, extensor pollicis brevis
Facet syndrome	muscles acting across the joint, e.g. rotatores, multifidi, semispinalis
Fibrositis (diffuse myofascial syndrome)	multisegmental; generally, muscles from cervical and lumbar nerve roots
Hallux valgus	extensor hallucis longus & brevis

Headaches:
  frontal
 	
  temporal
  vertex
  occipital
	
	upper trapezius, sternomastoid, occipitofrontalis
	temporalis, upper trapezius
	splenius capitis, cervicis
	suboccipital muscles

Idiopathic edema	lymphatic smooth muscles
Infrapatellar tendonitis	quadriceps femoris
Intervertebral disc (early stages)	muscles acting across the disc space, e.g. rotatores, multifidi, semispinalis

Syndrome	Shortened muscles
Juvenile kyphosis & scoliosis	unbalanced paraspinal muscles
"Low back sprain"	paraspinal muscles: e.g. iliocostalis lumborum & thoracis; also see "intervertebral disc"
Plantar fasciitis	flexor digitorum brevis, lumbricals
Piriformis syndrome	piriformis muscle
Rotator cuff syndrome	supra- & infraspinati, teres minor, subscapularis
"Shin splints"	tibialis anterior
Temporomandibular joint (TMJ)	masseter, temporalis, pterygoids
Tennis elbow	brachioradialis, extensor carpi ulnaris, extensor carpi radialis brevis & longus, extensor digitorum, anconeus

Table II. Segmental innervation of muscles 117

Table II. Segmental innervation of muscles

Segments in **bold type** are the primary innervating segments.

UPPER EXTREMITY

Muscle	Segmental innervation							
	XI	C3	C4	C5	C6	C7	C8	TI
Trapezius	**XI**	**C3**	**C4**					
Levator scapulae		**C3**	**C4**					
Rhomboideus minor & major			C4	**C5**	C6			
Latissimus dorsi					C6	**C7**	C8	
Pectoralis major					C6	**C7**	**C8**	TI
Serratus anterior				C5	**C6**	C7	C8	
Pectoralis minor							**C8**	TI
Deltoid			C4	**C5**	**C6**	C7		
Coracobrachialis				C5	**C6**	**C7**	C8	
Biceps brachii				**C5**	**C6**			
Teres major				**C5**	**C6**	C7		
Triceps brachii					C6	**C7**	**C8**	
Supraspinatus			C4	**C5**	C6			
Infraspinatus			C4	**C5**	C6			
Teres minor			C4	**C5**	C6	C7		
Brachialis				**C5**	**C6**			
Brachioradialis				**C5**	**C6**			
Pronator teres, flexor carpi radialis				C5	**C6**	C7		
Pronator quadratus					C6	C7	**C8**	TI
Palmaris longus					C6	**C7**	**C8**	TI
Supinator				C5	**C6**	C7		
Extensor carpi radialis brevis				C5	**C6**	**C7**	C8	
Extensor carpi				C5	**C6**	**C7**	C8	
Extensor carpi ulnaris, extensor digitorum					C6	**C7**	C8	
Extensor indicis, extensor digiti, minimi, extensor pollicis longus					C6	**C7**	**C8**	TI
Extensor pollicis brevis					C6	**C7**	C8	
Flexor carpi radialis					**C6**	**C7**	C8	

Muscle	Segmental innervation			
Flexor carpi ulnaris		C7	**C8**	**T1**
Palmaris longus	C6	**C7**	**C8**	T1
Flexor pollicis brevis, flexor digiti minimi brevis	C6	C7	**C8**	**T1**
Abductor pollicis	**C6**	**C7**	C8	T1
Flexor digitorum superficialis	C6	**C7**	**C8**	**T1**
Flexor digitorum profundus		C7	**C8**	**T1**
Flexor pollicis longus	C6	**C7**	**C8**	T1
Lumbricales, abductor pollicis brevis, abductor digiti minimi	C6	C7	**C8**	**T1**
Dorsal & palmar interossei			**C8**	**T1**
Opponens pollicis	**C6**	**C7**	**C8**	**T1**
Opponens digiti minimi		C7	**C8**	**T1**
Adductor pollicis			**C8**	**T1**

LOWER EXTREMITY

Muscle	Segmental innervation						
Pectineus	**L2**	**L3**	L4				
Tensor fasciae latae			**L4**	**L5**	S1		
Adductor brevis	L2	**L3**	**L4**	L5			
Rectus femoris, vastus lateralis, vastus medialis, vastus intermedius	L2	**L3**	**L4**	L5			
Sartorius	**L2**	**L3**	L4				
Adductor longus	L2	**L3**	**L4**				
Adductor magnus	L2	**L3**	**L4**	**L5**			
Gluteus maximus			L4	**L5**	**S1**	**S2**	S3
Semimembranosus			L4	**L5**	**S1**	S2	S3
Semitendinosus				**L5**	**S1**		
Biceps femoris			L4	**L5**	**S1**	**S2**	S3
Gluteus medius			**L4**	**L5**	**S1**	S2	
Gracilis	L2	**L3**	**L4**	L5			
Gluteus minimus			**L4**	**L5**	**S1**		
Quadratus femoris			**L4**	**L5**	S1		
Piriformis					**S1**	**S2**	S3
Gastrocnemius, soleus			L4	L5	**S1**	**S2**	S3
Flexor hallucis longus			L4	**L5**	**S1**	**S2**	S3
Flexor digitorum longus			L4	**L5**	**S1**	S2	
Peroneus longus & brevis			L4	**L5**	**S1**	S2	

Table II. Segmental innervation of muscles   119

Muscle	Segmental innervation			
Tibialis posterior	L4	**L5**	**SI**	S2
Tibialis anterior	**L4**	**L5**	**SI**	S2
Extensor digitorum longus	**L4**	**L5**	**SI**	S2
Extensor hallucis longus	**L4**	**L5**	**SI**	S2
Flexor hallucis brevis, flexor digitorum brevis		**L5**	**SI**	
Plantar & dorsal interossei			**SI**	**S2**
Extensor digitorum brevis	L4	**L5**	**SI**	S2

Sources of supplies

Although the author uses the following suppliers, you are encouraged to develop your own sources. Your local medical acupuncture society may be able to offer suggestions or recommendations.

Japanese needle plungers. I use Showa #6 from:

Nikka Industries Ltd.
611 Powell Street
Vancouver, BC
Canada V6A 1H2
Telephone: 001 604 251-2466
Fax: 001 604 251-7226

This plunger is made of chrome-plated brass. Although somewhat costly, it is durable and can last for years. The plunger requires cleaning and autoclaving (in paper purpose-use envelopes) after each use. You will need several plungers; the exact number depends on how many patients you treat per working session (I have 30 plungers). Make sure that you are not given a much cheaper plunger made of aluminium. I find they cannot accept a 2-inch needle, and the plungers do not last for long.

Stainless steel disposable acupuncture needles that fit the above plunger are available from:

AcuMedic Ltd
101–103 Camden High Street
London NW1 7JN
England
Telephone: 00 44 171-388 5783/
*   388 6704*
Fax: 00 44 171-387 5766

The AcuMedic needles are pre-sterilized and supplied in plastic tubes; by cutting both ends of the plastic tube a tubular guide is formed. Needles are available in:

50 mm, dia. 0.30 and 0.35 (2 inches) —most often used length.
30 mm, dia. 0.25 (1 inch)
15 mm, dia. 0.25 (½ inch)

Note: the thickness of their handles can be inconsistent; when they are too small, the needles tend to fall out of the Showa plunger. These needles are also available from Nikka Industries Ltd.

ITO ESS disposable needles are available from:

Electro-Therapeutic Devices Inc
570 Hood Road, Suite 14
Markham
Ontario
Canada L3R 4G7
Telephone: 001 416 494-7997/001
*   905 475-8344*
Toll Free (only in Canada): (800)
268-3834
Fax: 001 905 475-5143

Pre-sterilized (with ethylene oxide gas) stainless steel acupuncture needles supplied in blister packs without glass or plastic guides. Fit Showa plunger:

50 mm, dia. 0.25 or 0.30 (2 inches)
30 mm, dia. 0.25 or 0.30 (1 inch)

Needles for manual stimulation
AAA Stainless steel disposable

acupuncture needles for manual stimulation (with glass tubes). IMPORTANT: these needles, with glass tube guides, are used for manual stimulation. They are not intended for, and do not fit, the Showa #6 plunger.

AAA Acupuncture Inc
PO Box 44–45
Taipei
Taiwan
R.O.C.
Telephone: 00-886-2-725 1042
Fax: 00-886-2-725 2203

These needles are also available from Nikka Industries Ltd. Needle lengths available:

#2610	1 inch
#2612	1½ inch
#2614	2 inch
#2616	2½ inch
#2618	3 inch

(I use the 1-inch needle for the face, hand, elbow and neck. The 3-inch needle is useful for heavier patients, but it is also generally necessary for all patients for the buttock.)

TENS units
Most of the above suppliers also offer TENS units. I find the Pointer Plus—an inexpensive, hand-held acupuncture point-locator—easy to use to stimulate the inserted needle instead of twirling it. I also recommend the unit to patients for transcutaneous stimulation at home. The point-finder, powered by a 9 volt battery, can also provide galvanic stimulation:

Output intensity	0–22 mA
Frequency of output	10 Hz continuous
Pulse width	240 μs
Waveshape	biphasic square pulse with negative spike

Suggested reading

Basmajian J F, De Luca C J 1985 Muscles alive, their functions revealed by electromyography, 5th edn. Williams & Wilkins, Baltimore

Bradley W G 1974 Disorders of peripheral nerves. Blackwell Scientific, London

Cailliet R 1988 Soft tissue pain and disability. F A Davis, Philadelphia

Cailliet R 1988 Low back pain syndrome, 4th edn. F A Davis, Philadelphia

Chusid J G 1985 Correlative neuroanatomy and functional neurology, 19th edn. Lange Medical, California

Gunn C C Reprints on pain, acupuncture and related subjects. Available from the author.

Poland J L, Hobart D J, Payton O D 1981 The musculoskeletal system, 2nd edn. Medical Examination Publishing, New York

Sheon R P, Moskowitz R W, Bolber V M 1982 Soft tissue rheumatic pain: recognition, management, prevention. Lea & Febiger, Philadelphia

Travell J G, Simons D G 1983 Myofascial pain and dysfunction. The trigger point manual. Williams & Wilkins, Baltimore

Abbreviations for commonly treated muscles

In writing clinical notes, it is often convenient to use abbreviations for commonly treated muscles.

Upper extremity muscles	
Trapezius	TZ
Levator scapulae	LS
Rhomboideus minor & major	Rh mi & mj
Latissimus dorsi	Lat D
Pectoralis major & minor	Pect mj & mi
Deltoid	D
Coracobrachialis	CoBr
Biceps brachii	Bi
Teres major & teres minor	Teres mj & mi
Triceps brachii	TR
Supraspinatus	SS
Infraspinatus	IS
Brachialis	Brac
Brachioradialis	BrRad
Pronator teres	Pro teres
Flexor carpi radialis	Fl carp rad
Pronator quadratus	Pr quad
Palmaris longus	Plm lng
Supinator	Supin
Extensor carpi radialis	Ext carp rad
Extensor carpi ulnaris	Ext carp uln
Extensor digitorum	Ext dig
Extensor indicis	Ext ind
Extensor digiti minimi	Ext dig V
Extensor pollicis longus & brevis	Ext pol lng & brev
Flexor carpi ulnaris	Flx carp ul
Flexor pollicis longus & brevis	Flx pol lng & brev
Abductor pollicis & brevis	Abd poll & brev
Flexor digitorum	Flx dig

Upper extremity muscles

Abductor digiti minimi	Abd dig V
Dorsal interossei	Inteross
Opponens pollicis	Opp poll
Adductor pollicis	Add poll

Lower extremity muscles

Pectineus	Pect
Tensor fascia lata	TFL
Adductor brevis/longus/magnus	Add brev/lng/mag
Rectus femoris	Rect fem
Vastus lateralis/medialis/intermedius	Vast lat/med/inter
Sartorius	Sart
Gluteus maximus, medius, minimus	Glut max/med/min or GMM
Semimembranosus	Semimemb
Semitendinosus	Semitend
Biceps femoris	Bi fem
Gracilis	Grac
Quadratus femoris	Quad fem
Piriformis	Piri
Gastrocnemius	Gastroc
Soleus	Sol
Flexor hallucis longus	Fl hall lg
Flexor digitorum longus	Fl dig lg
Peroneus longus & brevis	Pero lg & brev
Tibialis posterior	Tib Post
Tibialis anterior	TA
Extensor digitorum longus	Ext dig lg
Extensor hallucis longus & brevis	Ext hal lg & brev
Flexor hallucis	Fl hal
Dorsal interossei	Inteross
Extensor digitorum brevis	Ext dig brev

Part 4

Appendices

List of appendices

Appendix 1   Neuropathic pain: a new theory for chronic pain of intrinsic origin. Annals of the Royal College of Physicians and Surgeons of Canada 22(5): 327–330, 1989 (summary) (With permission) **131**

Appendix 2   "Prespondylosis" and some pain syndromes following denervation supersensitivity. Spine 5(2): 185–192, 1980 (With permission from J. B. Lippincott Company) **133**

Appendix 3   Tenderness at motor points: a diagnostic and prognostic aid for low-back injury. Journal of Bone and Joint Surgery 58A(6): 815–828, 1976 (abstract) (With permission) **145**

Appendix 4   Tennis elbow and the cervical spine. Canadian Medical Association Journal 114: 803–809, 1976 (summary) (Reprinted from, by permission of the publisher, CMAJ 1976; 114) **147**

Appendix 5   Tenderness at motor points: an aid in the diagnosis of pain in the shoulder referred from the cervical spine. Journal of the American Osteopathic Association, 77: 196/75–212/91, 1977 (abstract) **149**

Appendix 6   Dry needling of muscle motor points for chronic low-back pain. A randomized clinical trial with long-term follow-up. Spine 5(3): 279–291, 1980 (abstract) (With permission from J. B. Lippincott Company) **151**

Appendix 7   Male pattern hair loss—a supraorbital nerve entrapment syndrome? International Journal of Acupuncture and Electro-therapeutic Research 5: 1980 (abstract) **153**

Appendix 8   Fibromyalgia—what have we created? Pain 60: 349, 1995 (With permission from Appleton and Lange, Norwalk, Connecticut, USA) **155**

Appendix 9   Questions commonly asked by patients **157**

The author and publishers have made every effort to trace the copyright holders for borrowed material. If they have inadvertently overlooked any, they will be pleased to make the necessary arrangements at the first opportunity.

Appendix I.
Neuropathic pain: a new theory for chronic pain of intrinsic origin

C. C. Gunn MA MB BChir
Annals of the Royal College of Physicians and Surgeons of Canada

SUMMARY

Why is acupuncture accepted in the East, especially for the treatment of chronic pain, but not in the West? One reason is that the modus operandi of acupuncture is not fully understood; another is the enigmatic nature of chronic pain. This article introduces a new concept of chronic pain, and suggests how acupuncture may relieve it.

Chronic pain may arise from sources that are extrinsic to the nervous system (for example, ongoing injury or inflammation), but it can also be intrinsic and the result of abnormal hypersensitivity (supersensitivity) in neuropathic or partially denervated structures. Neuropathic pain typically affects the musculoskeletal system, and a pivotal component of this type of pain is muscle spasm or shortening. Spasm can cause pain localised to muscle, but sustained muscle spasm or shortening mechanically overloads tendons and their attachments, and can produce pain in these structures.

Since neuropathic pain is different from nociception or inflammation, its treatment is also distinct (desensitization of super-sensitivity). Most physical treatment modalities for this type of pain, such as heat, massage or transcutaneous electrical nerve stimulation (TENS), desensitize by reflex stimulation of the affected part via its intact innervation. However these modalities are passive and limited in scope. Stimulation ends when their application is terminated. In contrast, injection techniques, including acupuncture, are more effective and long-lasting, because the tissue injury that they produce can unleash the body's healing source of bio-energy through the current of injury. Tissue injury also releases the platelet-derived growth factor (PDGF), which can promote healing.

Appendix 2.
"Prespondylosis" and some pain syndromes following denervation supersensitivity

C. C. Gunn MA MB BChir
Spine (From the Clinical Research Unit, Rehabilitation Clinic, Workers' Compensation Board of British Columbia, Richmond, British Columbia, Canada.
Presented in part at the 47th Annual Meeting of the Royal College of Physicians and Surgeons of Canada, January 27, 1978.)

SUMMARY

Pain is determined by the neurologic properties of receptor organs, neurons, and their interconnections. These may become supersensitive or hyperreactive following denervation (Cannon's Law). A common cause of denervation in the peripheral nervous system is neuropathy or radiculopathy as a sequel to spondylosis. Spondylosis in its early stage may be "asymptomatic" or painless and hence unsuspected, because small-diameter pain fibers may not initially be involved despite the attenuation of the other component fibers of the nerve. The term "prespondylosis" is introduced here to describe this presently unrecognized phase of insidious attrition to the other functions of the nerve, especially the trophic aspect. It is postulated that many diverse pain syndromes of apparently unrelated causation may be attributed to abnormal noxious input into the central nervous system from supersensitive receptor organs (nociceptors) and hyperreactive control systems at internuncial pools. Furthermore, trauma to a healthy nerve is usually painless or only briefly painful, unless there is pre-existing neuropathy. Some pain syndromes in muscle (e.g. trigger points and myofascial pain syndromes) and nerve (e.g. causalgia and diabetic neuropathy) that may be related to denervation are discussed.

Pain is merely an emotional response to afferent input; its perception is obviously influenced by emotion and dependent upon personality and mood. It is not a sensation in the strict neurophysiologic sense since there is no direct relation between the intensity of the applied stimulus and impulse-discharged frequency, nor between stimulus and the intensity of evoked experience. Yet, however complex the phenomenon of pain may appear to be, the flow of events from input of information into the nervous system (whether it be from a noxious or other stimulus) to final evoked response is determined by the neurobiologic properties of neurons and their interconnections.[43] All forms of adequate stimuli, both from the external world and from within the body, activate receptor organs. The information gathered by these receptor organs is transmitted to the central nervous system by way of primary afferent fibers. These synapse either directly on motoneurons or, more commonly, on interneurons. The latter may activate other interneurons in either the spinal cord or the brain. The patterns of interaction among these cells can be exceedingly complex. Eventually, however, the interneuron chains feed information to motoneurons, and these in turn command actions by effectors which include muscle and gland cells[43] (see Fig. 1).

This paper draws attention to the important but neglected role of supersensitivity of denervated structures[4] in the possible modification of afferent inputs and internuncial circuits. It is postulated that many diverse pain syndromes of apparently unrelated causation can probably be attributed to "denervation supersensitivity" and the development of hypersensitive receptor organs and/or hyperreactive control systems at internuncial pools. The concept of "prespondylosis", or the early pain-free

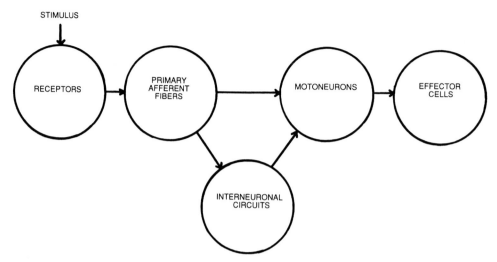

Fig. 1 Information flow in the nervous system. Receptors transmit information to the central nervous system via primary afferent fibers which synapse onto either motoneurons or interneurons. The latter may activate other interneurons, either in the cord or in the brain. Following complex patterns of interaction among these cells, information is fed to motoneurons and effector cells.

stage of spondylosis, as a cause of unsuspected peripheral neuropathy and denervation supersensitivity is introduced.

DENERVATION SUPER-SENSITIVITY[1,4,11,19,22,27,30,31,37]

Among the mysterious phenomena handed on from the physiologists of the 19th century to those of this century were two that were subsequently shown to have a common basis: the "paradoxical pupillary dilation"[4] and the "Philipeaux-Vulpian"[4] or "pseudomotor phenomenon".

It had first been noticed in 1855 that in an experimental animal, severance of the left cervical sympathetic nerve (preganglionic fibers) and simultaneous severance of the sympathetic branches above the right superior ganglion (post-ganglionic fibers) was followed by a curious difference in the two eyes: after approximately 48 hours the right pupil was larger than the left. Both irises had been deprived of their sympathetic connections, but the right pupil, deprived of its ultimate sympathetic nerve supply, was larger than the left, which was deprived of its penultimate supply.

The Philipeaux-Vulpian phenomenon described the anomalous response of denervated striated muscle to stimulation of nonmotor nerves distributed to adjacent blood vessels. It was noticed that when the hypoglossal nerve (motor nerve of the tongue muscles) was severed and allowed to degenerate, stimulation of the chorda tympani (sensory, vasodilator, and secretory fibers, but no motor fibers) caused the tongue to contract mysteriously.

It was not until many decades later that the explanation for these two mysteries was traced to the increased sensitivity of denervated structures to circulating transmitter agents. Denervation, it was shown, sensitized the retractor muscle of the iris to circulating adrenalin, causing the paradoxic exaggerated retraction on the denervated side. The pseudomotor phenomenon in the tongue occurred when the muscles, following denervation supersensitivity, responded to acetylcholine liberated at the terminals of the vasodilator nerve. Most of the early research was by Cannon and Rosenblueth,[4] who proposed a law of denervation (Cannon's Law), which stated, "When in a series of efferent neurons a unit is destroyed, an increased irritability to chemical agents develops in the isolated structure or structures, the effects being maximal in the part directly denervated". They showed that denervated striated muscle, smooth muscle, salivary glands, sudorific glands, autonomic ganglion cells, spinal neurons, and even neurons within the cortex develop supersensitivity.[4] Today, repeated animal experiments have confirmed that denervation supersensitivity is indeed a general phenomenon.[1,11,19,22,26,30,31,37] For example, in muscle, both striated and smooth, it has now been shown that there is an increase in the surface area of the muscle fiber that is sensitive to acetylcholine. Normally, the area of receptor sensitivity is very sharply circumscribed, but when the muscle loses its motor innervation there is a marked increase in the degree to which extrajunctional membrane responds to the application of acetylcholine. This change is detectable within a matter of hours and reaches a maximum in about a week, by which time the entire surface of the muscle fiber is as sensitive to acetylcholine as the normal end-plate region. This development of supersensitivity probably represents incorporation of newly synthesized receptors into extrajunctional membrane.

It is important to understand that actual physical interruption is not necessary for "denervation hypersensitivity" to develop. Minor degrees of damage or experimental exposure of motor axons to poisons such as colchicine or vinblastine can destroy the microtubules within the axons. Such a nerve still conducts nerve impulses, synthesizes and releases transmitted substances, and evokes both muscle action potentials and muscle contraction, but the entire membrane of the muscle cells innervated by the affected axon becomes supersensitive to the transmitter as if the muscle had been denervated. Destruction of microtubules within the axons is thought to disrupt axoplasmic flow and interfere with the trophic function of the nerve.

A second important change in muscle is the onset of spontaneous electrical activity of fibrillation. An innervated mammalian skeletal muscle normally gives an action potential only in response to the release of the transmitter agent. In contrast, action potentials begin to occur spontaneously within a few days after denervation and continue for as long as the muscle remains denervated, in some cases up to a year or more. This autogenic activity probably arises from local fluctuations in membrane potential and from an increase in membrane conduction to electrolytes. Other changes include those in muscle structure and biochemistry. Muscle atrophy eventually occurs following a progressive destruction of the fiber's contractile elements, resulting in a decrease in fiber diameter and slowing the speed of the contractile response. Another important but little understood change of denervated muscle fibers is a renewed ability to receive synaptic contacts. Unlike normal muscle fibers which resist innervation from foreign nerves, denervated muscle fibers accept contacts from a wide variety of sources, including other motor nerves, preganglionic autonomic fibers, and possibly even sensory nerves.

There are similar changes in neurons, but neurons are generally more difficult to investigate than muscle fibers because neuronal innervation is usually widely distributed on the soma and dendrites. Much of the early work also came from Cannon and his fellow workers, but it was not until the recent application of differential interference contrast microscopy (which allows visualization of living neuronal synapses) that sensitivity to acetylcholine was shown to be encountered at every point on the cell surface instead of only at the normal synaptic regions. Other effects of denervation on neurons have yet to be studied, but spontaneous activity of denervated sympathetic nerves has been described and has been suggested to be analogous to the fibrillation of denervated muscle fibers. As in muscle fibers, dener

136   **Appendices**

vation of neurons induces sprouting of nearby presynaptic elements, and nerve cells are more receptive to foreign innervation, with denervated autonomic neurons particularly prone to receive a variety of foreign synapses. Biochemical studies of peripheral neurons also show enzymatic changes following denervation, and it has been demonstrated that these too may affect the long-term regulatory mechanism in the peripheral and autonomic nervous systems.

Changes at synapses also occur. The studies of Hughes, Kosterlitz, and others[20,21,34] have shown that endogenous morphine-like peptides (endorphins and enkephalins) inhibit neuronal activity by altering sodium conductance at opiate receptors in the brain and at the spinal cord levels. Methionine-enkephalin is a neurotransmitter found in spinal gray matter occurring at the terminals of interneurons. Excitation of these interneurons, which interact with one another and impinge on the nerve endings of sensory neurons, produces primary afferent depolarization or presynaptic inhibition and attenuates nociceptive transmission across the synapses of primary afferent fibers and second order neurons, especially in Laminae I, II, and III. Chronic lesions of the primary afferents decrease the number of opiate receptors in the dorsal horn with a corresponding reduction of interneuron activity and presynaptic inhibition by enkephalin. Peripheral nerve disease may therefore also cause facilitation of noxious inputs at the dorsal horn.

PERSISTENT PAIN FOLLOWING NEUROPATHY AND DENERVATION

The simple idea of a closed chain of neurons producing an invariable response when stimulated is no longer tenable, yet the fundamental physiologic fact remains that once an action potential is initiated in a receptor organ by a threshold stimulus, it is propagated to the central nervous system by way of primary afferent

neurons that synapse either directly on motoneurons or, more commonly, on interneurons. It is the pattern of interaction among interneurons and multineuronal assemblies[33] in the spinal cord and in the brain that can be exceedingly complex, modifying the message on its way to the brain, possibly diverting it into other pathways or suppressing it completely.[43]

Three basic concepts have been formulated to explain the peripheral encoding of painful stimuli. These are (1) *intensity* coding, (2) the *pattern* theory, and (3) the *specificity* hypothesis. Despite arguments to the contrary, the evidence is compelling that some receptors (nociceptors) and neurons are at least relatively specialized to signal stimuli of tissue-damaging intensity. However, because excitation of receptors other than nociceptors can contribute to the sensation of pain, a modified polymodal pattern concept has also been proposed. Nociceptors consist of the terminations of thinly myelinated Group Aδ (Group III) fibers, diameter 1–4 mm and conducting at 5–45 meter/sec ("fast pain"), and C (Group IV) non-myelinated fibers, which are thinner and conduct at about 1 meter/sec ("slow pain"). These fibers synapse with neurons in the dorsal horn and are relayed via interneurons to higher centers, probably with control systems to regulate the input of noxious stimuli at several levels. Because supersensitivity occurs as a general phenomenon following denervation, heightened neuronal and interneuronal activity may exist throughout the nervous systems—peripheral, central, and autonomic.

In the peripheral nervous system, a common cause of neuronal destruction is peripheral neuropathy when there is disordered function and/or structure of the peripheral nerve. While the causes of peripheral neuropathy are many and varied (congenital, neoplasms, inflammatory, traumatic, vascular, toxic, metabolic, infective, degenerative, idiopathic, and others), the peripheral nerve responds with only a limited repertoire of pathologic reactions.[2] This may be either attenuation of the caliber of axons or primary damage to myelin, but is usually a combination of both. Variable degrees of damage with variable degrees of reversibility may be present, ranging from neurapraxia to axonotmesis and neurotmesis.[32,36] Peripheral neuropathy may occur at various sites, but the spinal root within the spinal canal and intervertebral foramina, and even after it emerges, is especially prone to damage.[2,42] This may follow acute trauma, but more usually it is the long-term sequela of spondylosis which causes simultaneous damage to the nerve roots (radiculopathy) and cord (myelopathy).[42] Spondylosis (which refers to the structural disintegration and morphologic alterations in the intervertebral disc and pathoanatomic changes in surrounding structures) has been acknowledged as a clinical entity only for some 20 years,[42] although even today the significance of the silent, pain-free, but not necessarily morbidity-free, prespondylotic phase is still not widely recognized. "Prespondylosis" may be "symptomless", its symptoms and signs unsuspected, because pain may not be a feature. Pain occurs only when and if the degenerative changes impinge upon local pain-sensitive structures to produce local pain, or upon pain fibers of the nerve root to produce the transmitted pain of "radiculitis", a clinical term commonly used to describe the discomfort or pain radiating along the peripheral nerve. However, constant attrition of the peripheral nerve can attenuate fibers other than those of pain (which are small and less liable to mechanically caused ischemia),[43] producing insidious neuropathy, the effects of which are projected onto the dermatomal, myotomal, and sclerotomal target structures supplied by the segmental nerve. Dysfunction may be motor, sensory, trophic, or autonomic,[12] but since pain fibers are not necessarily involved, there are no "symptoms" and both patient and physician may be oblivious to the condition. "Prespondylosis" nonetheless has its implications

and may contribute to chronic pain. For example, whereas acute structural deformation of a healthy nerve is not painful or only briefly so (e.g. peroneal nerve palsy[8] or radial nerve "Saturday night" palsy), such is not the case in an unhealthy nerve. It has recently been shown that when and if pain develops in a peripheral nerve, it is primarily associated with the acute breakdown of myelinated fibers (either Wallerian or axonal degeneration) superimposed on the pre-existence of chronic nerve fiber degeneration.[10] Pain is probably not caused simply by the different proportions of large to small fibers remaining after nerve degeneration as anticipated by the gate theory, but by the acute upon chronic or recent abnormal rate of breakdown of myelinated fibers (whatever its primary cause may be).[10] Animal experiments have furthermore shown that an acute mechanical injury to a healthy dorsal nerve root does not produce a sustained discharge unless there has been pre-existing minor chronic injury to the nerve.[39] Clinically, it is also common knowledge that in asymptomatic subjects the mere appearance of degenerative changes in spinal roentgenograms is not of much clinical significance, but in these persons, disability after injury will tend to be prolonged and signs of radiculopathy more commonly found.[13,14] It would therefore appear that for pain to persist after trauma, a prerequisite is the existence of chronic nerve irritation.

DENERVATION SUPERSENSITIVITY AND MYALGIC HYPERALGESIA

Myalgic hyperalgesia, or excessive tenderness to digital pressure, is not a normal feature of muscle because their mechanosensitive nociceptors are located deep within the muscle bulk and have high thresholds. (Muscle Aδ fibers are mechanosensitive, have high thresholds, and respond to strong localized pressure but not to stretch or ischemia. Muscle C fibers also have high mechanical thresholds but in addition are excited by ischemia combined with contraction of the muscle.) Myalgic hyperalgesia may be *local* or traumatic following local injury and tissue damage when algogenic chemical substances such as 5-hydroxy-tryptamine, histamine, bradykinin, and hydrogen ions are liberated. These produce an unspecific but powerful excitatory effect on nociceptors as well as on those low-threshold mechanoreceptors that have myelinated afferent fibers.[44] Myalgic hyperalgesia may also be *secondary* to neuropathy when the nociceptors develop supersensitivity following denervation. Tenderness is then maximum at the neurovascular hilus where nociceptors are most abundant around the principal blood vessels[43] and nerves as they enter the deep surface of the muscle to reach the muscle's motor zone of innervation. As this zone is fairly constant in position for each muscle,[6,7] tenderness in muscles secondary to neuropathy is easily found. Tenderness at the muscle's zone of innervation is often loosely referred to as *at* the "motor point"[41] (a point on skin where a muscle twitch may be evoked in response to minimal electrical stimulation). Variable degrees of tenderness at motor points are usually present in the upper and lower limb muscles of persons who have some degree of spondylotic radiculopathy, the degree of myalgic hyperalgesia paralleling the radiculopathy.[13,15] The presence of tenderness at motor points within an affected segmental myotome is therefore a useful diagnostic and prognostic aid following spinal injuries.[12-15]

In some cases of denervation supersensitivity it may be possible for the afferent barrage from muscle nociceptors (at the zone of innervation and musculo-tendinous junctions) and their connections via spinal interneurons to become self-perpetuating, thus constituting, in effect, a "trigger zone or point".[16,24,27,38] A comparison of the maps of trigger points produced by Travell and Rinzler[38] with that of motor points will show their spatial coincidence. Furthermore, trigger zones may be demonstrated to coincide with motor points by electrical stimulation.

Many painful conditions that are presently labeled as vague clinical entities ("tendinitis", "bursitis", or "fibrositis") are probably hyperalgesic nociceptor regions in myofascial structures. For example, in midcervical spondylosis, tenderness at the anterior deltoid muscle motor point and the bicipital tendon is called "bicipital tendinitis".[14] Tenderness at the wrist extensor muscle motor points and musculotendinous junctions around the lateral epicondyle of the elbow is commonly called "tennis elbow" or "lateral epicondylitis"[14] (the tenderness at the bony epicondyle is probably sclerotomal). Myalgic hyperalgesia in the left pectoral muscles has been mistaken for angina and cardiac pain. "Bursitis" around the hip is not an uncommon diagnosis, yet surgical intervention rarely reveals a bursa distended with serous fluid. This "bursitis" is often tender gluteal muscle motor points secondary to lumbar spondylosis.[17] These entities presently saddled with diverse, non-descript labels may be demonstrated by electrical stimulation to be motor points, and electromyography will generally show electrodiagnostic evidence of radiculopathy,[13,14] but even simple palpation can reveal hyperalgesia in the several muscles supplied by both anterior and posterior primary rami (i.e. at root level) within the same segmental level or myotome.[18] In these conditions, treatment should logically be addressed to the underlying spinal problem; in our experience, this has been followed by resolution of symptoms.[12–14]

Supersensitivity of denervated structures may also lead to muscle spasm which is so often a co-feature of pain.[12] Muscle tone may be increased at the muscle spindle whose intrafusal fibers, innervated from higher centers by the gamma motoneurons, may be subjected to increased impulse traffic. Hypersensitivity of the primary and secondary endings, which are sensitive to stretch of the central portion of the spindle, may also overstimulate the essential feedback mechanism by which skeletal muscle and resting muscle tonus are controlled. The afferent discharge of the spindle via the dorsal root on the motoneurons of the same muscle is excitatory.

DENERVATION SUPER-SENSITIVITY AND NEURALGIC HYPERPATHIA

The extreme example of causalgia is discussed first, as its manifold manifestations represent all aspects of peripheral neuralgic hyperpathia. The term "causalgia" is derived from the Greek kausis, "burning", and algos, "pain", to describe the most striking feature of the condition, which is persistent, severe, and burning pain in an affected extremity, usually as the result of a partial injury to a nerve (commonly, the median, ulnar, and sciatic nerves).[9,26,35] In addition to the pain there is invariably autonomic dysfunction and trophic changes in skin and/or bones in the involved part. Causalgic pain has been categorized as "major causalgia" and a less painful variant referred to as "minor causalgia" or "posttraumatic reflex sympathetic dystrophy". Typically, causalgic pain appears within a week following a nerve injury (when denervation supersensitivity has had time to develop), but its onset may be delayed by as much as 3 months. The severe, burning pain may be explained by hypersensitivity of receptors and small-diameter afferent fibers ($A\delta$ and C) in cutaneous and other tissues. The autonomic dysfunction and trophic changes may likewise be the result of supersensitivity at lateral horn cells, autonomic ganglia, and receptors around blood vessels; thus, a sympathetic nerve block and/or sympathectomy provides relief in a proportion of patients.

Doupe and co-workers[9] have suggested that trauma causes the formation of "artificial synapses" (ephapses) between sympathetic efferents and somatic sensory afferent nerves. According to this theory, a sympathetic impulse traveling down the efferent nerve, in addition to its usual effects, causes depolarization of the somatic sensory nerve at the point of artificial synapse. This depolarization is then propagated orthodromically along the afferent sensory nerve and when added to normal sensory impulses causes abnormally high sensory discharge which is felt as pain. In addition, depolarization at the artificial synapse is said to propagate antidromically along the somatic afferent, leading to the release of certain substances[5] that decrease the threshold at the sensory nerve ending and further increase the impulses reaching central areas.

Livingston's[25] theory of the "vicious cycle of reflexes" postulated that there is chronic irritation of a peripheral sensory nerve leading to increased afferent impulses and resulting in abnormal activity in an "internuncial pool" of neurons in the lateral and anterior horns of the spinal cord. The concept of denervation supersensitivity supports Livingston's theory, because peripheral receptors, afferent neurons, internuncial pools, and autonomic ganglia may become hypersensitive or hyperreactive. Furthermore, autonomic neurons may generate spontaneous autogenic potentials similar to muscle fibrillations (see above). However, the increased receptivity of denervated autonomic neurons to a variety of foreign synapses and peripheral nociceptors to released algogenic substances[5] also supports the theory of artificial synapses proposed by Doupe and co-workers. It is also significant that changes at spinal and other central synapses may occur (see above) with facilitation of noxious input.

In recent years the well-known gate theory of Melzack and Wall[28] has been applied to causalgia (and to many other pain syndromes). It is suggested that cells in the substantia gelatinosa of the dorsal horn of the spinal cord act as a "gate control system", modifying the transmission of afferent sensory impulses. This theory emphasizes a pattern of impulses rather than single impulses with a "selection process" to explain the intricacies of sensory experience. The gate theory contends that impulses from large myelinated fibers inhibit or "close the gate", whereas tonic background impulses transmitted along smaller fibers (which include afferent sympathetic fibers) "open the gate" to facilitate transmission. The theory also proposes a descending control system originating in the brain that modulates the excitability of afferent conduction. The "gate theory", published in 1965, was written before the present explosion of information about the anatomic state of nerves in the peripheral neuropathies. Wall and Melzack were influenced, in particular, by a study on postherpetic neuralgia in which it was shown that intercostal nerve biopsy specimens had a preferential loss of large myelinated fibers, and Noordenbos[29] had generalized from this observation to propose that pain was a consequence of a loss of inhibition normally provided by the large fibers. It is now known that loss of large fibers is not necessarily followed by pain.[10] In many conditions (e.g. Friedreich's ataxia) there may be a large-fiber deficit without pain. Wall, now realizing that any attempt to correlate the remaining fiber diameter spectrum with pain is no longer possible, has restated the gate control theory of pain recently[40]:

1. Information about the presence of injury is transmitted to the central nervous system by peripheral nerves. Certain small-diameter fibers (Aδ and C) respond only to injury while others with lower thresholds increase their discharge frequency if the stimulus reaches noxious levels.
2. Cells in the spinal cord or fifth nerve nucleus that are excited by these injury signals are also facilitated or inhibited by other peripheral nerve fibers that carry information about innocuous events.
3. Descending control systems originating in the brain modulate the excitability of the cells that transmit information about injury.

Therefore the brain receives messages about injury by way of a gate-controlled system that is influenced by (1) injury signals, (2) other types of afferent impulse, and (3) descending control.

In this restatement, Wall stated that fiber diameter alone is not enough or is even completely irrelevant to explain pain in the neuropathies when pathologic peripheral fibers have unusual impulse generation and conduction properties. However, the original proposal that transmission of information about injury from the periphery to the first central cells is under control (influenced by peripheral afferents and by descending impulses), still holds. In denervation supersensitivity, as mentioned above, facilitation of noxious input may occur at the "gate" in the dorsal horn from a reduction of presynaptic inhibition through interneurons. This facilitation may also occur at autonomic ganglia where interneurons have been described.

Because the peripheral nerve responds with only a limited repertoire to the many and varied causes of neuropathy,[2] it is to be expected that other forms of neuropathy and neuralgic hyperpathia (whatever their primary cause) will have many common features. For example, in diabetic neuropathy,[3] the unremitting pain, characteristic cutaneous hypersensitivity, burning sensations, paresthesias, and autonomic symptoms are certainly not specific for diabetes. Histologic findings in nerve biopsy specimens have indicated that the diabetic lesions are predominantly in the small fibers, with nerve sprouting (a feature of denervation supersensitivity) the likely cause of the pain.

DISCUSSION

An enigma in the past, and today a source of great interest to neurobiologists, the importance of denervation supersensitivity with regard to pain has not been appreciated. The implications of Cannon's Law of denervation are probably far more embracing than the few conditions briefly discussed here. It is possible that many other forms of pain, e.g. trigeminal or postherpetic (neuralgic) and even chronic low back pain, are a post-denervation supersensitivity phenomenon rather than the result of noxious stimuli. Thus, pain may be the central perception of (1) an afferent barrage from noxious stimuli or (2) the abnormal input into the central nervous system from ordinarily non-noxious stimuli rendered excessive through overly sensitive receptors (or a variable combination of both). Consider, therefore, the chronic "low back" patient whose discomfort still persists following resolution of the acute phase. Though not crippled or even in distress, he is unable to cope with any but light activities. Such a patient may not be subjected to noxious stimuli (nociception) but may be "hyperalgesic" in that ordinarily non-noxious stimuli, e.g. prolonged standing, sitting, or walking, can cause symptoms. "Pain" as a scientific term should preferably be discarded and a distinction made between "nociception" and "hyperalgesia", because different approaches are required in their management. A source of nociception should be eliminated— an unstable fracture or spondylolisthesis stabilized, the unrelenting spatial compromise of an impinging disc or carpal tunnel relieved, or the inflammatory and algogenic agents of trauma soothed. In hyperalgesia, any contributory factors from spinal spondylosis should be alleviated (traction, support, mobilization, or even surgery) and the hypersensitive structures desensitized. Lomo[26] has shown in animal experiments that denervation supersensitivity (as assayed by the sensitivity of muscle extrajunctional membrane to acetylcholine) may be reduced or abolished by electrical stimulation. The analgesic effect of transcutaneous neural stimulation may thus depend in part on the reduction of supersensitivity as on the neurohumoral inhibitory effects of the spinal and brainstem antinociceptor systems. Continuous stimulation was found most effective, and it has been suggested that the efficacy of needle acupuncture for hyperalgesia may be due in part to stimulation by the current of injury.[18]

Supersensitivity in autonomic pathways can furthermore lead to the increased blood vessel tone of virtually all tissues and cause secondary pain by structural disintegration. Following denervation, the total collagen in soft and skeletal tissues is reduced. Replacement collagen also has fewer cross-links and is markedly weaker than normal mature collagen.[23] Because collagen provides the strength of ligaments, tendons, cartilage, and bone, this may contribute to many degenerative conditions in the weight-bearing (spinal and intervertebral disc) and activity-stressed parts of the body (tendinitis, cuff tears, epicondylitis, ruptured tendons, and so forth). These secondary conditions, presently dignified by various terms to imply specific clinical entities, are probably only the ultimate sequelae of neuropathy. Degenerative disc disease itself may not be a primary condition. The structural integrity, strength, and reparative capacity of these somatic tissues are such that the constant wear of normal usage is probably adequately compensated for, unless their trophic capability is depressed, as in chronic neuropathy. Thus, in a young person the supraspinatus tendon does not rupture but avulses from its bony insertion, and the intervertebral disc (now thought to be the prime causative factor in spondylosis) is so strong that following violence to the vertebral column, the bones always give way first. The disc is particularly vulnerable to altered vascular tone, being almost avascular and dependent largely upon diffusion through adjacent spongy bone for nutrition. It is food for thought that in all our recent studies,[12–15] early and subtle signs of peripheral neuropathy were found in a significant number of young (under 30 years), apparently normal, and asymptomatic subjects. Prespondylosis, a term introduced here to describe the early effects of spondylotic attrition on the peripheral nerve, is generally painless, though not necessarily devoid of morbidity. It and its frequent companion, radiculopathy, would therefore seem to be fertile areas for further study in order to understand better the genesis of pain and "degenerative" conditions.

REFERENCES

1. Axelsson J, Thesleff S: A study of supersensitivity in denervated mammalian skeletal muscle. J Physiol 174: 178, 1959
2. Bradley W G: Disorders of Peripheral Nerves. Oxford, Blackwell Scientific Publications, 1974, pp 129–201, 253–267
3. Brown M J, Martin J R, Asbury A K: Painful diabetic neuropathy. Arch Neurol 33: 164–171, 1976
4. Cannon W B, Rosenblueth A: The Supersensitivity of Denervated Structures. New York, The Macmillan Company, 1949, pp 1–22, 185
5. Chapman L F, Ramos A O, Goodell H, Wolff H G: Neurohumoral features of afferent fibres in man. Arch Neurol 4: 617–650, 1961
6. Coers C: Note sur une technique de prelevement des biopsies neuro-musculaires. Acta Neurol Psychiatr Belg 53: 750–765, 1953
7. Coers C, Woolf A L: The technique of muscle biopsy. Chap 1. The Innervation of Muscle. Oxford, Blackwell Scientific Publications, 1959, pp 1–41
8. Denny-Brown D, Brenner C: Paralysis of nerve induced by direct pressure and by tourniquet. Arch Neurol Psychiatry 51: 1–26, 1944
9. Doupe J, Cullen C H, Chance G Q: Post-traumatic pain and causalgic syndrome. J Neurol Neurosurg Psychiatry 7: 33–48, 1944
10. Dyck P J, Lambert E H, O'Brien P C: Pain in peripheral neuropathy related to rate and kind of nerve fibre degeneration. Neurology 26: 466–477, 1976
11. Fambrough D M, Hartzell H C, Powell J A, Rash J E, Joseph N: On differentiation and organization of the surface membrane of a post-synaptic cell—the skeletal muscle fibre, Synaptic Transmission and Neuronal Interaction. New York, Raven Press, 1974, pp 285–313
12. Gunn C C, Milbrandt W E: Early and subtle signs in "low back sprain". Spine 3: 267–281, 1978
13. Gunn C C, Milbrandt W E: Tenderness at motor points—a diagnostic and prognostic aid for low-back injury. J Bone Joint Surg 58A: 815–825, 1976
14. Gunn C C, Milbrandt W E: Tennis elbow and the cervical spine. Can Med Assoc J 114: 803–809, 1978
15. Gunn C C, Milbrandt W E: Tenderness at motor points—an aid in the diagnosis of pain in the shoulder referred from the cervical spine. JAOA 77: 196/75–212/91, 1977
16. Gunn C C, Milbrandt W E: Utilizing trigger points. The Osteo-Physician, March 1977, pp 29–52
17. Gunn C C, Milbrandt W E: "Bursitis" around the hip. Am J Acupuncture 5: 53–60, 1977
18. Gunn C C, Milbrandt W E: Dry needling of muscle motor points for chronic low-back pain: A randomized clinical trial with long-term follow-up. Spine (In press)
19. Guth L: "Trophic" influences of nerve on muscle. Physiol Rev 48: 645–687, 1968
20. Hughes J, Smith T W, Kosterlitz H W, et al: Identification of two related pentapeptides from the brain with potent opiate agonist activity. Nature 258: 577–579, 1975
21. Hughes J, Kosterlitz H W, Smith T W: The distribution of methionine-enkephalin and leucine-enkephalin in the brain and peripheral tissues. Br J Pharmacol 61: 639–647, 1977
22. Katz B, Miledi R: The development of acetylcholine sensitivity in nerve-free segments of skeletal muscle. J Physiol 170: 389–396, 1964
23. Klein L, Dawson M H, Heiple K G: Turnover of collagen in the adult rat after denervation. J Bone Joint Surg 59A: 1065–1067, 1977
24. Kraus H: Triggerpoints. NY State J Med 73: 1310–1314, 1973
25. Livingston W H: Pain Mechanism. Physiological Interpretation of Causalgia and Its Related States. New York, The Macmillan Company, 1943
26. Lomo T: The role of activity in the control of membrane and contractile properties of skeletal muscle. Chap 10. Motor Innervation of Muscle. Edited by S Thesleff. London, Academic Press, 1976
27. Melzack R, Stillwell D M, Fox E J: Trigger points and acupuncture points for pain—correlation and implications. Pain 3: 3–23, 1977
28. Melzack R, Wall P D: Pain mechanisms: A new theory. Science 150: 971–979, 1965
29. Noordenbos W: Pain. Amsterdam, Elsevier, 1959
30. Purves D: Long-term regulation in the vertebrate peripheral nervous system. Chap 3. International Review of Physiology. Neurophysiology II, Vol 10. Edited by R Porter. Baltimore, University Park Press, 1976, pp 125–177
31. Rosenblueth A, Luco J V: A study of denervated mammalian skeletal muscle. Am J Physiol 120: 781–797, 1937
32. Seddon H J: Three types of nerve injury. Brain 66: 237–288, 1943
33. Shepard G M: Microcircuits in the nervous system. Sci Am 238: 93–103, 1978
34. Snyder S H: Opiate receptors in the brain. N Engl J Med 296: 266–271, 1977

35. Sternschein M J, Myers S J, Frewin D B, Downey J A: Causalgia. Arch Phys Med Rehabil 56: 58–63, 1975

36. Sunderland S: Nerve and Nerve Injuries. Edinburgh, E & S Livingstone, 1968

37. Tower S S: The reaction of muscle to denervation. Physiol Rev 19: 1–48, 1939

38. Travell J, Rinzler S H: The myofascia genesis of pain. Postgrad Med 11: 425–434, 1952

39. Wall P D, Waxman S, Basbaum A I: Ongoing activity in peripheral nerve injury discharge. Exp Neurol 45: 576–589, 1974

40. Wall P D: The gate control theory of pain mechanisms—a re-examination and re-statement. Brain 101: 1–18, 1978

41. Walthard K M, Tchicaloff M: Motor points. Chap 6. Electrodiagnosis and Electromyography. Third edition. Edited by S Licht. Baltimore, Waverly Press, 1971, pp 153–170

42. Wilkinson J: Cervical Spondylosis—Its Early Diagnosis and Treatment. Philadelphia, WB Saunders Company, 1971, pp 1–8

43. Willis W D, Grossman R G: Medical Neurobiology. St. Louis, CV Mosby Company, 1973, pp 1–4, 53, 71

44. Zimmerman M: Neurophysiology of nociception. Chap 4.[30] pp 79–221

Appendix 3.
Tenderness at motor points: a diagnostic and prognostic aid for low back injury

C. C. Gunn MA MB BChir and W. E. Milbrandt MD
Journal of Bone and Joint Surgery (From the Workers' Compensation Board, Rehabilitation Clinic, Vancouver)

ABSTRACT

In patients with low back injury the motor points of some muscles may be tender. Of fifty patients with low back "strain", twenty-six had tender motor points and twenty-four did not, while forty-nine of fifty patients with radicular signs and symptoms suggesting disc involvement had tender motor points, and the one without such tender points had a hamstring contusion which limited straight leg raising. Of fifty controls with no back disability, only seven had mild tender points after strenuous activity, while forty-six of another fifty controls with occasional back discomfort had mild motor-point tenderness. In all instances the tender motor points were located in the myotomes corresponding to the probable segmental levels of spinal injury and of root involvement, when present.

Patients with low back strain and no tender motor points were disabled for an average of 6.9 weeks, while those with the same diagnosis but tender motor points were disabled for an average of 19.7 weeks, or almost as long as the patients with signs of radicular involvement, who were disabled for an average of 25.7 weeks. Tender motor points may therefore be of diagnostic and prognostic value, serving as sensitive localizers of radicular involvement and differentiating a simple mechanical low back strain from one with neural involvement.

Appendix 4.
Tennis elbow and the cervical spine

C. C. Gunn MA MB BChir and W. E. Milbrandt MD

Canadian Medical Association Journal (From the Workers' Compensation Board, Rehabilitation Clinic, Vancouver)

SUMMARY

The exact cause of tennis elbow, a common condition, is still obscure. While the condition may well be entirely due to a local disorder at the elbow, the results of a study of 50 patients whose condition was resistant to 4 weeks of treatment directed to the elbow suggest that the underlying condition may have been (at least in these patients) a reflex localization of pain from radiculopathy at the cervical spine. Clinical, radiologic, and electromyographic findings supported this suggestion. The pain was demonstrated to be muscular tenderness, which was maximal and specific at motor points. Treatment directed to the cervical spine appeared to give relief in the majority of patients. The more resistant the condition, the more severe were the radiologic and electromyographic findings in the cervical spine.

Appendix 5.
Tenderness at motor points: an aid in the diagnosis of pain in the shoulder referred from the cervical spine

C. C. Gunn MA MB BChir and W. E. Milbrandt MD

Journal of the American Osteopathic Association

ABSTRACT

Cervical spondylosis, a universal degenerative condition, often is misdiagnosed, because it causes no symptoms unless it impinges on pain-sensitive tissues or a nerve root to cause radiculitis and consequently is difficult to detect in early stages. It is possible to recognize neuropathy, however, by the presence of tenderness at motor points, since spondylotic pain may be transmitted via the segmental nerve to the corresponding myotome and felt as muscle pain and tenderness, which may be elicited easily at the motor point. In a combination prospective/retrospective study of 407 patients with primary shoulder pain, 50 patients who showed no obvious physical signs required electromyography for definitive diagnosis. Observations of tender motor points in these patients are compared with the medical records of the remaining 357 patients. Tender motor points were always found in patients with cervical spondylosis and shoulder pain, but absent in patients with extrinsic shoulder pain unless accompanied by concurrent spondylosis.

Appendix 6.
Dry needling of muscle motor points for chronic low back pain.
A randomized clinical trial with long-term follow-up

C. C. Gunn MA MB BChir, W. E. Milbrandt MD, A. S. Little MD and K. E. Mason BSc MSc

Spine (From the Workers' Compensation Board, Rehabilitation Clinic, Vancouver)

Fifty-six male patients who had chronic low back pain of at least 12 weeks' duration (average duration, 28.6 weeks) and who had failed to respond to traditional medical or surgical therapy were entered into a randomized clinical trial to compare the relative efficacies of the Clinic's standard therapy regimen with and without dry needling at muscle motor points. Before entering the trial, all patients had undergone without improvement eight weeks of the Clinic's standard therapy regimen of physiotherapy, remedial exercises, and occupational therapy. The 29 study subjects and 27 control patients then continued with this regimen, but the study subjects also received needling at muscle motor points once or twice a week (average number of treatments, 7.9). All patients were assessed at the time of discharge, 12 weeks after discharge, and at the time of writing (average, 27.3 weeks). The group that had been treated with needling was found to be clearly and significantly better than the control group ($P > 0.005$, N = 53) with regard to status at discharge, status at 12 weeks' follow-up, and status at final follow-up. At final follow-up, 18 of the 29 study subjects had returned to their original or equivalent jobs and 10 had returned to lighter employment. In the control group, only four had returned to their original work and 14 to lighter employment; nine were still disabled. The results seem to justify the procedure in chronic low back patients in whom myofascial pain (the majority) rather than skeletal irritation is the dominant disabling feature.

Appendix 7.
Male-pattern hair loss—a supraorbital nerve entrapment syndrome?

C. C. Gunn MA MB BChir and Mathew H. M. Lee MD MPH FACP
International Journal of Acupuncture and Electro-therapeutic Research

The cause of male-pattern hair loss remains obscure. It is noted to occur in the geographic distribution of the supra-orbital and sometimes the great occipital nerves. It is suggested that these nerves are susceptible to entrapment and subsequent neuropathy since signs of the latter precede and accompany hair loss. Male-pattern alopecia is uncommon in women, yet neuropathy and deprivation of the trophic factor can lead to hair loss in any part of the body in both men and women. It seems therefore that scalp hair loss, more common in the male, occurs because higher levels of testosterone create a situation in which scalp nerves become vulnerable to neuropathy. Testosterone greatly increases muscle and skeletal bulk, thickens skin and reduces subcutaneous fat, most especially in the head. These factors may well cause increased tension to scalp nerves.

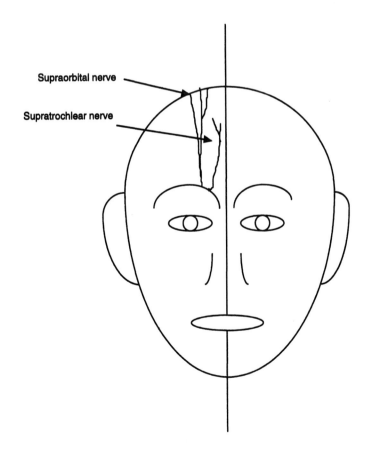

Supraorbital nerve

Supratrochlear nerve

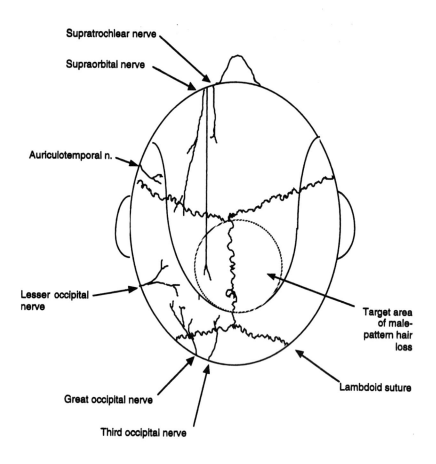

Supratrochlear nerve

Supraorbital nerve

Auriculotemporal n.

Lesser occipital nerve

Target area of male-pattern hair loss

Lambdoid suture

Great occipital nerve

Third occipital nerve

Appendix 8.
'Fibromyalgia'—"What have we created?"

C. C. Gunn MA MB BChir
Pain

'Fibromyalgia' has recently become a popular diagnosis and many doctors now apply the American College of Rheumatology (ACR) 1990 criteria for the classification of fibromyalgia. Regrettably this has brought hopeless despair to countless individuals. I have witnessed many patients who suffer from chronic musculoskeletal pain designated and treated as 'fibromyalgia'. However when their pain failed to respond to popular fibromyalgia treatment (such as tricyclic medications) they were abruptly abandoned as the condition is commonly viewed as a life-time disorder even worthy of life-long compensation.

The ACR criteria have been promoted as highly sensitive and specific, but for what condition? Far from being a distinctive syndrome fibromyalgia merely describes the most extreme and extensive of the mundane aches, pains and tender muscles that we all have in various degrees at one time or other. For example, mildly tender points are not unusual in asymptomatic individuals, especially after strenuous physical activity, and moderately tender points are not exceptional in those who have a history of a 'vulnerable' spine. These subjects although asymptomatic characteristically have minor degenerative changes visible on roentgenograms.

Tender sites are almost consistently found in muscle at motor points or at muscle–tendon junctions. (One ACR designated location is in a pad of fat although fatty tissue is not well endowed with pressure receptors.) Patients with myofascial pain invariably have multiple tender points and even in localized conditions, such as lateral epicondylitis, examination will reveal numerous tender sites scattered throughout the body in a myotomal disposition—to practiced fingers, the number of tender sites in a fibromyalgic patient can be many times the stipulated number.

Many physicians who treat musculo-skeletal pain disregard the term 'fibromyalgia' or 'fibrositis' preferring to use 'myofascial' pain and identifying the specific muscles and spinal level(s) that are involved. At a recent symposium on fibromyalgia it was allowed that fibromyalgia cannot be distinguished from myofascial pain (and the putative association with sleep disturbance not proven).

Patients with widespread myofascial pain should unfailingly be given a competent and comprehensive examination of the musculoskeletal system. This examination must include careful palpation of individual muscles for tenderness, increased tone and muscle shortening (e.g. taut muscle bands, enthesopathic tendons, restricted joint range).

The examination is never complete without the evaluation of deep muscles especially the intrinsic muscles of the back (e.g. the semispinalis and multifidus muscles). These muscles, generally beyond the reach of a probing finger, can only be explored by using a dry-needling technique.

Fibromyalgia has not been shown to be caused by ongoing nociception or inflammation, and psychologic factors have been ruled out. Its many features (such as widespread aching, point tenderness, skin fold tenderness, articular pain, swelling of the hands or knees, numbness or coldness of the extremities, reticular skin discoloration, irritable bowel and trophedema) suggest a functional and/or structural alteration in the peripheral nervous system.

For instance, tenderness is usually escorted by other manifestations of radiculopathy and the most significant of these is muscle shortening. Shortened muscles are diffusely present in axial as well as in limb musculature; although they can produce muscle ache and pain by compressing intramuscular nociceptors, they can also produce pain by pulling upon tendons and ligaments. However, most significantly, shortening of paraspinal muscles can compress the intervertebral disc and irritate the nerve root to create a vicious circle that can perpetuate the problem.

It is naive and unkind to condemn a patient solely because of a few tender points. A patient with chronic musculo-skeletal pain deserves a complete and competent physical examination. Whenever a physical examination is inconclusive, needle exploration of deeper muscles must be resorted to, because an unwarranted diagnosis that is based only on tender points can grievously delay or deter appropriate treatment.

It is worth retelling that effective treatment for myofascial pain is available; patients with myofascial pain improve significantly when painful and shortened muscle bands are released by the dry-needle technique of Intramuscular Stimulation (IMS).

Appendix 9.
Questions commonly asked by patients

I wish he would explain his explanation
        BYRON: DEDICATION TO DON JUAN

Q: I have been in many clinics to treat my aching back and legs. I have had many medical investigations including X-rays. I have tried physiotherapy, manipulations, and pills without any lasting relief. My doctors tell me they have found nothing wrong. But why are my "aches and pains" still with me and so difficult to treat? Is surgery necessary?

A: Pain is not one entity but three. Type One is well known and easily understood. There is an obvious painful cause from injury. Think of a burn on the skin, or a cut from a knife. Type Two pain is the pain of inflammation, such as a sprained ankle when there is obvious swelling, redness and the ankle is hot to touch. These two types of pain and their treatment are well understood by the medical profession.

Since an obvious cause of pain from injury or inflammation has not been found, it is very likely that there is no actual source of pain. This is not unusual; the pain you feel is caused by abnormal and excessive sensitivity of your body's nervous system. This is medically known as "supersensitivity". Unfortunately, supersensitivity has received little attention in medical circles. Since there is no pain source, surgery will not help and is definitely not indicated.

Q: If my pain is Type Three, what makes my nerves supersensitive?

A: The basic problem is that the nerves going to your painful area are unwell. Doctors call it neuropathy. Unwell nerves behave abnormally—they are too sensitive; they tend to magnify ordinary inputs and change them into painful sensations. Supersensitivity usually occurs when there is some irritation to the nerve roots that come from your spinal cord. Probably your nerves were already weakened (through wear and tear, or aging), and it took only a minor accident to trigger them into supersensitivity.

Q: How can my supersensitive nerves be treated?

A: Supersensitivity cannot be operated on and "cut away", but it can be desensitized. "Pain killers" and other pills only mask pain briefly. What your nerves need is energy to heal themselves. That is why we instinctively massage a painful part to provide mechanical energy and to revitalize it. Heat—or thermal energy—is another commonly used form of treatment. In fact, all effective treatments for Type Three pain are different forms of energy.

Q: But I've tried massage and heat. They only give me temporary relief. Why?

A: All types of local treatment have their limitations. They cannot penetrate deeply into the body and the duration of their energy input is temporary. For instance, the energy of a massage does not last much longer than the massage itself. That is why I prefer to use a needle treatment that is a modification of traditional acupuncture. A needle causes a minute local injury, and the injury does two important things. Firstly, the injury generates electrical energy (as proven by Galvani over 300 years ago), and muscle spasm is released. The injury also releases fresh blood into the painful site and blood platelets have a healing effect. The needle's main purpose is not to block pain (although it does this too), but to stimulate the body to heal itself. It's as close to a "cure" as you can get.

Q: I've heard of acupuncture and that it can help pain. How is Intramuscular Stimulation different?

A: Acupuncture is an ancient philosophy and its diagnosis and practice in Traditional Chinese or Oriental Medicine are not based on modern science. What was a great approach 4000 years ago can be improved with today's medical knowledge. Intramuscular Stimulation or IMS relies on neurology and a Western understanding of anatomy for diagnosis and treatment.

Q: I've always been nervous about needles. Is it painful?

A: The acupuncture needle is very fine—much finer than the hollow needle used to inject medicine or to take a blood sample. You may not even feel its penetration through the skin, or if you do, it's only a mild and momentary prick. If your muscle is normal, the needle inside you is painless. However, if your muscle is supersensitive and in spasm, and if the needle is correctly placed, you'll feel a peculiar sensation—like a charleyhorse or muscle cramp. This is a distinctive type of discomfort, caused by the muscle grasping the needle. Patients soon learn to recognize and welcome it. They call it a "good" or positive pain because it quickly disappears and is followed by a wonderful feeling of relief and relaxation. The needle may still be in you, but because the muscle is no longer tight, you don't feel it anymore. Therefore, the needle itself is painless. What has happened is that the needle has caused your abnormal muscle spasm to be intensified briefly, and then released. It is important that you experience this peculiar sensation in order to have relief.

Q: But some of my friends tell me they have had painless acupuncture and have not felt these sensations.

A: Many doctors perform traditional acupuncture by inserting needles into locations according to acupuncture "maps". They are not seeking the epicenter of the painful muscle. Sometimes they may add electrical stimulation to the inserted needles. This type of acupuncture is not so painful—but the results may not be as good as IMS.

Q: How long will the benefit last?

A: The effects of IMS are cumulative. Each needle injury stimulates a certain amount of healing, until eventually, the condition is healed and the pain disappears. Blood also brings a healing factor, known as the platelet derived growth factor, to injured tissues. IMS is like pruning a plant: you produce small injuries to stimulate new growth to replace injured tissues. But once healing has occurred, you are back to where you were before the pain occurred.

Q: How often are treatments necessary?

A: Treatments are usually once a week because time is needed between treatments for the body to heal itself. Also, stimulation for healing remains for several days, lasting for as long as the injuries caused by the needle are present. Treatment can be spaced out to two weeks.

Q: How many treatments will I need?

A: The number of treatments depends on several factors: your general health, the duration and extent of your condition, how much scar tissue there is—previous surgery is bad news—and how quickly your body can heal. The rate of healing also depends on the condition of your nerves; young people usually heal quicker, but older is not necessarily slower. If the pain is of recent origin, one treatment may be all that is necessary. In my published study of patients with low back pain, the average number of treatments required was 8.2.

Q: Does IMS always succeed?

A: There is no absolute guarantee, but if the diagnosis of nerve supersensitivity pain is correct, and the part of the body requiring treatment is capable of healing, then the probability of healing should be the same as that for a cut in your finger.

Treatment fails if the diagnosis is wrong, or treatment improperly applied. IMS, of course, has no effect on structural defects, such as in late osteoarthritis when there has been severe bone erosion.

.

Index

Abbreviations, commonly treated muscles, 125–126
Achilles tendonitis, 99, 100–101
Acquired immunodeficiency syndrome (AIDS), 37
Adductor tubercle, 91, 92
Adson's maneuver/test, 43
Anterior thigh and knee, 91–96
Anxiety states, 32, 58
Appendices, 127–159
Autonomic changes, 26
Autonomic manifestations of neuropathy, 8–9
Autonomic (segmental) reflexes, 76–78
see also Reflex stimulation

Back, 41–42, 75–86
tender motor points as a diagnostic and prognostic aid, 145
Back pain, 13, 16, 28, 75–76, 83
Bicipital tendonitis, 7, 11
Bursitis, 29, 115
ischial, 89
pre-patellar, 115
trochanteric, 89
Buttock, 87–89

Calcaneal heel spur, 103
Calf, 99–101
Cannon and Rosenblueth's law of denervation, 5–6, 85
Capsulitis, shoulder, 66
Carpal tunnel syndrome, 4, 29, 71–72
Cautions, 37
Cervical fibrositis, 14
Cervical spine, 42, 44, 51–60
shoulder pain, 149
tennis elbow, 147
Choice of needles, 32–33, 83
Chondromalacia patellae, 28, 96
Chronic pain summary, 23
Cluster headache, 58, 59
Collagen degradation, 9–10
Collagen formation, 9
Contraindications, 37
Costoclavicular maneuver/test, 43

De Quervain's disease (tenosynovitis), 28, 71
Degenerative joint disease, 72
Denervation, Law of, 5–6, 85
Deqi phenomenon, 12–13
Diagnosis, guidelines for, 25–29
Dorsal back, 75–78
Dry needling, 11, 31
low back pain clinical trial, 18, 151
Dupuytren's contractures, 73

Edema, 9
see also Trophedema
Elbow and forearm, 12, 66–71
Electrical stimulation, 12, 35–36
Electromyography, 5, 7, 9, 33
Epicondylitis, 13, 14, 28, 70, 71, 147
Examination, general, 15, 39–46
Examination, regional
see also Regional examination and treatment
anterior thigh and knee, 91–92
buttock, 89
calf, 99–100
cervical spine, 51–54
dorsal back, 75–76
elbow and forearm, 66–70
foot, 101
leg and dorsum of foot, 96–98
lumbar back, 78–82
posterior thigh, 90
shoulder, 61–63
wrist and hand, 71

Fabere (Patrick's) test, 44, 92
Facet (joint) syndrome, 7
Fascia lata fasciitis, 89
Fibrositis (Fibromyalgia), 8, 13–15, 32, 36, 155–156
Fibrotic contractures, treatment of, 13, 85–86
Finding points, 33–34
Finding spasm, 34–35
Foot, 101–103
see also Leg and dorsum of foot
Frozen shoulder, 66

General examination, 15, 39–46

Hair loss, 9, 27, 153
Hallux rigidus, 102
Hallux valgus, 29, 101
Hammer lock test, 58, 62–63
Headache
cluster, 58, 59
migraine, 58, 59
muscle contraction (tension), 59
Hepatitis, 37
HLA-B27 spinal arthropathies, 93
Human immunodeficiency virus (HIV), 37

Iliotibial band friction syndrome, 89
Inflammation, 3, 23, 31
Intramuscular stimulation (IMS), 11–16
Invisible lesion, 16
Ischial bursitis, 89

Knee, examination and treatment, 91–96
Knee pain, 94–96
Knee, structural problems, 96

Lasegue's sign, 43–44
Lateral epicondylitis, 7, 14, 28, 70
Law of denervation, 5–6, 85
Leg and dorsum of foot, 96–99
Leg lengths, 40
Longstanding disorders, 13
Low level laser therapy (LLLT), 36
Lower limb, 87–103
Lumbago, 83
Lumbar back, 78–86

Matchstick test, 9, 26, 73
Medial epicondylitis, 71
Metatarsalgia, 102
Migraine headache, 58, 59
Mishaps, 37
Morton's (plantar) neuralgia, 102–103
Motor manifestations of neuropathy, 4, 5, 26–27
Muscle contraction (tension) headache, 59
Muscle shortening, 6–7, 10, 11, 15–16, 17, 26, 28–29, 109, 111
see also General examination; Regional examination
common syndromes (table), 115–116
Muscles
Abductor digiti minimi, 102
Abductor hallucis, 102
Abductor pollicis, 71
Abductor pollicis brevis, 72
Abductor pollicis longus, 68
Adductor brevis, 92
Adductor hallucis, 102
Adductor longus, 91, 92
Adductor magnus, 92
Adductors, 32, 91, 92, 102
Anconeus, 67, 70
Biceps brachii, 11, 68
Biceps femoris, 90, 94
Brachialis, 68
Brachioradialis 67, 68, 70
Coracobrachialis, 68
Deltoid, 63, 65, 66
Erector spinae, 12, 28, 52, 84
Extensor carpi radialis brevis, 67, 70
Extensor carpi radialis longus, 67, 70
Extensor carpi ulnaris, 67, 70
Extensor digiti minimi, 67, 70, 73
Extensor digitorum, 67, 70, 73
Extensor digitorum brevis, 97
Extensor digitorum longus, 97, 100, 102

Muscles (*contd*)
  Extensor hallucis brevis, 101
  Extensor hallucis longus, 97, 101,
    102
  Extensor indicis, 68, 73
  Extensor pollicis brevis, 68
  Extensor pollicis longus, 68, 71
  Flexor carpi radialis, 69, 71
  Flexor carpi ulnaris, 69, 71
  Flexor digiti minimi, 102
  Flexor digiti minimi brevis, 102
  Flexor digitorum brevis, 102
  Flexor digitorum longus, 28, 100,
    101, 102
  Flexor digitorum profundus, 28,
    69, 73
  Flexor digitorum sublimis, 69, 71
  Flexor digitorum superficialis, 73
  Flexor hallucis brevis, 102, 103
  Flexor hallucis longus, 100, 101,
    102
  Flexor pollicis brevis, 72
  Flexor pollicis longus, 69
  Gastrocnemius, 99
  Gluteus maximus, 28, 87, 88
  Gluteus medius, 41, 48, 88, 94
  Gluteus minimus, 48, 88
  Gracilis, 91, 95
  Iliocostalis cervicis, 53, 81
  Iliocostalis lumboram, 81, 84
  Iliocostalis thoracis, 81
  Iliopsoas, 91
  Infraspinatus, 63, 64, 65, 66
  Interossei, 72, 73, 102
  Latissimus dorsi, 52, 62, 64, 65,
    75, 81, 84
  Levator labii superioris, 59
  Levator scapulae, 52, 53, 54, 57,
    58, 62, 63, 64, 75, 81
  Longissimus capitis and cervicis,
    52, 53, 54, 55, 58, 81, 85
  Lumbricals, 103
  Multifidius, 82
  Obliquus externa, 84
  Opponens digiti minimi, 118
  Opponens pollicis, 72
  Palmaris longus, 69, 71
  Paraspinal, 7, 15–16, 27, 31, 48,
    56, 109
  Pectineus, 91
  Pectoralis major, 65–66
  Pectoralis minor, 66
  Peroneus brevis, 98, 100
  Peroneus longus, 98, 100
  Peroneus tertius, 97
  Piriformis, 87, 93–94
  Popliteus, 94, 100
  Pronator quadratus, 29, 69, 71,
    72
  Pronator teres, 29, 69, 71, 72
  Pronators, 29, 69, 71, 72
  Quadratus femoris, 48, 88
  Quadratus lumborum, 84
  Quadratus plantae, 103

Quadriceps femoris, 11, 16
Rectus femoris, 95
Rhomboids, 52, 62, 63, 64, 75
Rotatores, 82
Sacrospinalis, 81
Sartorius, 91, 94–95
Scalenus, 53, 54, 57
Semimembranosus, 90, 95
Semispinalis, 51, 53, 54–55, 58, 82
Semitendinosus, 90, 95
Soleus, 36, 99
Splenius capitis and cervicis, 52,
  53, 54, 55, 56, 57, 58, 59, 81
Sternomastoid, 53, 54, 55, 57
Subscapularis, 63, 66
Supinator, 68, 70
Supraspinatus, 57, 63–64
Teres major, 63, 64, 65, 66
Teres minor, 63, 64, 66
Tibialis anterior, 11, 36, 97, 100
Tibialis posterior, 100, 101
Trapezius, 32, 37, 51, 52, 53, 54,
  55, 56–57, 58, 62, 64, 75, 81
Triceps brachii, 68, 70
Vastus intermedius, 95
Vastus lateralis, 95
Vastus medialis, 95
Myofascial pain, 3–4, 6, 7, 8, 9, 14,
  15, 32

Needle, choice of, 32–33, 83
Needle holder, 11
Needle technique, 11–12, 31–38
Needle-grasp 12, 13, 16, 17, 34
Neurometer, 33–34, 35
Neuropathic, muscle, 7, 33
Neuropathic pain
  clinical features of, 3–4, 5
  intrinsic origin, 131
Neuropathic pain, definition of 3, 5
Neuropathic pain and neuropathy,
  3–10
Neuropathy, causes, of 4–5
Neuropathy, manifestations of,
  25–27
Neuropathy pain model, 107–112
Nociception, 3, 23

Pain in the
  back, 13, 16, 28, 75–76, 83
  back of the knee, 100
  calf, 100
  dorsal region, 75–76
  elbow joint, 12, 68
  epicondylar region, 70–71
  foot, medial aspect, 101
  groin, 92
  knee, 11, 16, 94–96
  lateral elbow, 67–68
  medial elbow, 69–70
  patellofemoral, 96
  pubis, 92–93

  sole, 102–103
  wrist, 73
Patellofemoral pain, 96
Patient questions, 157–159
Patrick's sign, 44
Piriformis syndrome, 93–94
Plantar fasciitis, 103
Plantar (Morton's) neuralgia,
  102–103
Point-finder, using, 33–34, 35
Points, 33–35
Posterior thigh, 90
Precautions, 37
Prespondylosis, 133–141

Questions, patient, 157–159

Radial pulses, 43
Radiculopathy, 3–10, 23, 43
Radiculopathy, features of, 25
References
  Part 1: 18–19
  Part 4: 142–143
Reflex stimulation, 12–13, 17–18,
  111
  see also Autonomic (segmental)
    reflexes
Regional examination and
  treatment, 47–103
Release of muscle spasm and
  shortening, 12, 31, 35–36
  see also Regional examination
Releasing vasospasm, 18
Rheumatoid arthritis, 3, 73
Rosenblueth and Cannon's Law of
  denervation, 5–6, 85

Sacroiliac joint, 93
Segmental innervation of muscles
  (table), 117–119
Segmental involvement, 27–29
Sensory manifestations of
  neuropathy, 25
Shin splints, 11, 98
Shortened muscles in common
  syndromes (table), 6–7
Shoulder, 42, 61–73
  referred pain, cervical spine, 149
Side effects, 37, 54, 57
Sign
  Fabere (Patrick's), 44, 92
  Lasegues's, 43–44
  Trendelenburg's, 41
Sources of supplies, 121–122
Spasm, 6–7, 12, 33, 34, 35, 56
Specific treatment, regional
  examination and, 47–103
Spinal arthropathies, 93
Spondylolisthesis, 29
Spondylosis, 4–5, 10, 25, 107–112
Super-contractures, 85–86

Supplies, sources of, 121–122
Supraorbital nerve entrapment
    syndrome, 153–154

"Teh Ch'i" phenomenon, 12–13
Temporomandibular joint (TMJ),
    59–60
Tender motor points as a
    diagnostic and prognostic aid,
    low back injury, 145
Tendonitis, 7, 28
Tennis elbow see Epicondylitis
Tenosynovitis, 28, 71, 100
Tensor fasciae latae, 28

Test
    Combined modified Adson's
        and costoclavicular, 43
    Fabere (Patrick's), 44, 92
    Hammer lock, 58, 62–63
    Lasegue's sign, 43–44
    Matchstick 9, 26, 73
    Skin rolling, 26
    Trendelenburg's sign, 41
Thigh, 90–94
Tibial stress syndrome, 98–99
Tic douloureux (Trigeminal
    neuralgia), 59
Transcutaneous electrical nerve
    stimulation (TENS), 12, 35–36

Treatment goals, 31–32
Trigeminal neuralgia (Tic
    douloureux), 59
Trigger finger, 28, 72
Trigger points, 7, 26, 109
Trochanteric bursitis, 89
Trophedema, 9, 16, 26, 51

Upper limb, 42, 44, 61–73

Vasovagal reaction 37, 54, 57

Whiplash syndrome, 58
Wrist and hand, 71–73

Edwards Brothers Malloy
Thorofare, NJ USA
January 4, 2013